The Little
HELMET MAN
or Cranio-What?

The Little
HELMET MAN
or Cranio-What?

Foreword by Neurosurgeon Dr. David F. Jimenez, M.D. &
Plastic surgeon Dr. Constance M. Barone, M.D. the pioneers of
minimally invasive Endoscopic Strip Craniectomy

TATIANA TURNER

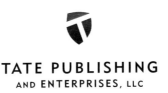

TATE PUBLISHING
AND ENTERPRISES, LLC

Published by Tate Publishing & Enterprises, LLC
127 E. Trade Center Terrace | Mustang, Oklahoma 73064 USA
1.888.361.9473 | www.tatepublishing.com

Tate Publishing is committed to excellence in the publishing industry. The company reflects the philosophy established by the founders, based on Psalm 68:11,
"The Lord gave the word and great was the company of those who published it."

Book design copyright © 2012 by Tate Publishing, LLC. All rights reserved.
Cover design by Jan Sunday Quilaquil
Interior design by Jake Muelle
Illustrations by Lenka Korbelics

Published in the United States of America

ISBN:978-1-62510-976-7
1. Medical / Surgery / Neurosurgery
2. Biography & Autobiography / Personal Memoirs
12.11.01

Dedication

I dedicate this book to Dr. David F. Jimenez, neurosurgeon, and his wife, Dr. Constance M. Barone, plastic surgeon—the couple with very special skills and an unbelievable combination of professionalism, humanity, and endless, sincere love for their little patients.

Foreword by Dr. David F. Jimenez and Dr. Constance M. Barone

Soon after we met for the first time in our surgical residency, we realized that we had a strong passion and fervor for treating infants and children, particularly those affected with craniofacial disorders. Concurrent to our lifetime commitment to each other, we decided to concentrate our efforts, passion, and skills to treating children with craniosynostosis and related conditions. Craniofacial surgery offers the operating surgeons a wide array of surgical procedures that are challenging, complex, demanding, and yet, very rewarding.

To take a baby's skull almost completely off and then reconstruct it to normalcy is indeed technically rewarding and satisfying. Yet when we crossed the line to parenthood, we found ourselves at the other end of the spectrum. If we had a baby with craniosynostosis, would we let him or her go through such an experience?

Our techniques had improved from taking seven-to-nine hours per case to an average of 3.1 hours. Our blood transfusion rate decreased from 100 percent to sixty-seven percent. Who would we allow to operate on our expected child? As it turned out, he was perfect and without the need for intervention. Yet that experience propelled us to reconsider the options. Could the surgery be done less invasively? Could we decrease the need for blood transfusions? Could we minimize the amount of trauma sustained by the baby and decrease hospitalization time? Finally, could we improve the final long-term results and outcomes as compared to the traditional surgery we were performing? The answer, as it turned out sixteen years later, is a resounding yes!

We still remember the day that Patrick and his parents came to meet us for the first time. They had done their homework and research. A decision was made to travel from California to the far away state of Texas and consult with doctors they had never met to hand over their most precious possession to complete strangers. We met and spoke for a long time, answered all their questions, and placed their minds and souls at ease (perhaps harder to do than the surgery itself). With trust and faith in their hearts, they handed him over to us for treatment. Surgery was a complete success. It lasted forty-one minutes, he lost a tablespoon of blood, and Patrick was discharged from the hospital the next morning.

This book eloquently depicts the journey of one of our almost 600 surgical patients. It describes the angst, apprehension and disquietude that parents often experience when facing an unknown diagnosis, conflicting treatment modalities and attempting to make the best decision for their baby. It tells a compelling story of hope, faith and trust. As it turns out, Patrick is now a very handsome, bright, intelligent young man who looks absolutely normal and remembers nothing of what happened to him years ago.

We applaud Mrs. Turner for writing her story for others to learn and benefit. Who knows, maybe someday, Patrick will advance to the field of his choice to ultimately help humanity and others around him.

Dr. David F. Jimenez
Dr. Constance M. Barone
June 2012

Craniosynostosis.

Try saying that word three times fast. The word is a mouthful, and it is as scary as it is long. I wasn't a young mother at all, and Patrick wasn't my first child. Despite this, I didn't have a clue that something like craniosynostosis existed. I also didn't have the knowledge that craniosynostosis runs in my husband's family…until it happened to our baby.

Doctors always say to keep an eye on your baby's head. I wasn't a first-time mother, so I already knew to keep my eyes on the big soft spot on the top of the head.

I knew the soft spot has a diamond shape, which should not close too early or too late.

But I didn't know to pay attention to the other cranial sutures, bumps, or ridges all around the baby's head. *What is a cranial suture*? I would have thought.

When I started to mother Patrick, I knew something was amiss. His head wasn't the same as other children's and definitely not the same as his siblings' heads when they were his age. I attributed Patrick's narrow head to my husband's side of the family with their longer foreheads. "He doesn't have a forehead. He has a fivehead," we teased. Patrick was our endearing little alien.

Even though we acted lighthearted, our baby's condition was still unsettling.

Every night, I kissed Patrick's fivehead. Hair will eventually cover it up. I comforted myself. But, day-by-day, his head lengthened. It will stop growing longer, right?

I was wrong. Wrong and completely unaware of what was actually at work here.

Craniosynostosis is an unfamiliar term to most mothers. I myself read "What to Expect" books religiously to ensure that I had awareness of what could potentially befall my precious infant. Craniosynostosis can be genetic, as is the case for our family. But *any* baby is at risk—even if this condition hasn't occurred in your family before.

My greatest hope for this book is that parents understand the basic information about proper baby skull formation. I also hope to raise awareness of skull abnormalities that can occur with any infant. Emergencies never happen at a convenient time. Parents desperately want to believe that their babies won't experience any complications during their growth, but it is very possible. We need to accept this and acquaint ourselves with the risks.

Our dear Patrick did have craniosynostosis. Whenever you hear that your child has an unwanted condition, it feels like somebody threw a bag of bricks in your gut. You're shocked. You're numb. You're unable to process the information. *My child…has what? No. It cannot be true.* The shock waves turn into waves of pain and desperation. You know that you're all the child has. You have to be strong for the child and find a solution immediately. Finding the solution consumes your waking hours.

Thankfully for us, Dr. Jimenez walked into our life with this highly desired solution. We knew Patrick would need surgery. The idea of knives and foreign instruments contacting and opening his body ached our hearts. Dr. Jimenez understood our fear but quickly assuaged them. He explained his unique procedure that almost guaranteed success. For his work with our child, we are forever grateful.

To aspiring doctors or doctors in training: I cannot stress enough how invaluable Dr. Jimenez's work is to the medical world. He pioneered endoscopic/less invasive surgery for craniosynostosis patients. The evolution of craniosynostosis treatment is a long and troubled road. In the previous century, infant mortality rates were high. Even if the child lived through the risky procedure, complications were common and dangerous. But nowadays because of Dr. Jimenez, once-concerned parents can sleep soundly at night knowing that their babies are in deft hands. This less invasive procedure puts less stress on the babies' bodies (and less stress on the parents). Train yourselves; learn from Dr. Jimenez. Your patients will have a greater peace of mind with his method compared to the harsh treatments of passed years.

Again, this book is dedicated to Dr. Jimenez and his wife, Dr. Barone. You change lives everyday with your passionate work. My son could not have been in more caring, masterful hands. He's now a normal kid, and you'd never know he went through any major surgery at all.

Part One
Lessons on Craniosynostosis

Chapter 1
ABC of Infant's Skull Anatomy

❧

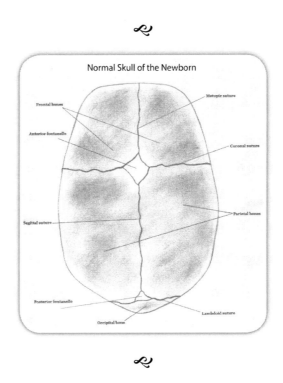

Normal Skull of the Newborn

Metopic suture

Frontal bones

Anterior fontanelle

Coronal suture

Parietal bones

Sagittal suture

Posterior fontanelle

Lambdoidal suture

Occipital bone

❧

B efore parents can spot abnormalities in their children's skulls, they must know what a healthy skull looks like.

For parents to be aware of a healthy skull, it is important to learn its different sections. Consult the picture above for a corresponding visual.

An infant's skull is made up of several bones:

- ❑ Two *frontal bones,* which build the front of the skull.
- ❑ Two *pariental bones*, which build the largest part of the skull—the top, sides, and back.
- ❑ One *occipital bone* in the lower-rear section of the head.

Typically, the cranial bones remain separate until about age two. The cranial bones are held together by strong, fibrous tissues called *cranial sutures*. In infants, cranial sutures are very flexible. This is helpful in allowing the head to pass through the birth canal during delivery.

As the brain grows, these sutures stretch and produce new bone, allowing the skull to grow into a normal adult shape, along with the underlying brain. These are the different types of sutures:

Vertical sutures

- ❑ *The metopic suture* extends to the forehead, between the soft spot and the upper bridge of the nose.
- ❑ *The saggital suture* is the longest suture, which goes from the soft spot on the top to the back of the head.

Horizontal sutures

❑ *The coronal suture* extends from the soft spot on the top of the head to an area in front of the left or right ear.

❑ *The lambdoid suture* is located at the back of the head.

Spaces between the bones within the fibrous tissues are called *fontanelles*. The fontanelles should feel flat and firm. A bulging fontanel is often a sign of increased pressure within the brain. The fontanelles bulge in a crying or vomiting infant but should return to normal when the infant is calm. Sunken fontanelles are a sign of an infant's dehydration. This can result from sicknesses that involve diarrhea or vomiting; so the parents should look for sunken fontanelles when their baby experiences these problems. Be wary of a sunken fontanelle—this can be a medical emergency and require immediate treatment.

❑ *Big fontanelles* on the top of the head are in the shape of a diamond. This is also called the "soft spot," which usually closes between seven and nineteen months. You can often see this structure pulsating like a heartbeat.

❑ *Small fontanelles* are in the back of the head, in the shape of triangle, and usually close by the time an infant is one to two months old.

❑ *Two small fontanelles* are by the ear area on both
   sides of the head.

❧

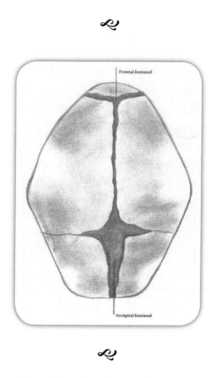

❧

These fontanelles close by themselves as part of normal
growth. I, as most mothers, knew about the diamond-
shaped fontanel and knew that I can feel my baby's
heartbeat by gently touching on the top of the soft spot.

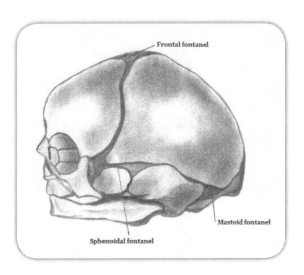

But what about the rest of the head?

I was never told to look for ridges or other bumps along the baby's head, which could reveal signs of a serious problem. The brain grows rapidly in the first year of the baby's life. A full-term baby is born with forty percent of his adult brain volume. This increases to eighty percent by age three. Thanks to the skull sutures, which hold the baby's skull bones together, the brain is able to expand while being protected.

If one or more of these sutures close prematurely, the brain has no room to expand in that area. So it expands in different directions, and the head shape becomes deformed. For instance, if the sutures close at the top of the head, the sides of the head expand, or the sides may be closed and so the head grows longer and longer, as Patrick's. When this happens, the condition called Craniosynostosis occurs.

Chapter 2
Cranio-*what*?

Every time I asked people the question—and I asked a lot—if they were familiar with Craniosynostosis, I consistently heard the same answer: "Cranio-*what*?"

It didn't matter whom I asked: parents, aunts, uncles, and even people working or studying in the medical field. I experienced the horrifying reality check—people have zero knowledge that conditions like craniosynostosis exist. It didn't surprise me because I was one of those people who didn't know anything about this condition. The word "craniosynostosis" wasn't in my vocabulary…until it happened to my son. If somebody had asked me the same question back then, he or she would have received the same answer from me: "Cranio-*what*?" Understand that I wasn't a first-time, inexperienced mother. Patrick was my third child. By that time, I had read a metric ton of books about pregnancy and the baby's life throughout the first years—*none* mentioned anything about this condition. It was like a fantasy, like it didn't exist.

When we first met with Dr. Jimenez the day before Patrick's surgery, I already did some speedy homework about Craniosynostosis and browsed website after website to better understand what the heck it was. All I knew was that it had too many syllables and it sounded like a scary word. I tried to organize every bit of information in my head, but I became very overwhelmed with all the medical terms. Sutures? Saggital sutures? Fontanelles? I was already exhausted from what hit us so suddenly, and as hard as I tried to become better acquainted with the topic in such a short time, I did not do a good job. I tried to read and study, but my attempts always ended up with me staring at the pictures of babies' heads posted on various websites. I didn't want to believe that our son's head shape looked the same as the craniosynostosis patients'. It was heartbreaking. But I must tell you after our first meeting with Dr. Jimenez, there was not a single thing I couldn't understand. His explanation was absolutely perfect, very understandable, and I finally understood what was going on here.

Based on Dr. Jimenez's easy-to-follow discussions with us, here is a basic overview of craniosynostosis to answer the most common questions.

What is craniosynostosis, exactly?

"Craniosynostosis is a congenital deformity of the infant skull that occurs when the fibrous joints between the bones of the skull (called cranial sutures) close prematurely." As one would expect, this causes the head to grow abnormally, becoming deformed and misshapen. This barricades the brain from growing naturally and may present dangerous complications if not treated within the first few months of an infant's life. This includes neurological and cognitive problems because the brain can't expand in the directions it needs to.

According to the various types of suture closures, there are different types of synostosis, or synthesis. These vary in degree of severity and subsequent treatment. Unlike other types of head malformations, craniosynostosis has a distinct and recognizable head shape that separates it from other possible conditions quickly. Depending on environmental factors and the abnormality present, head malformations can and often do fix themselves. It is important to note that everyone has a unique head shape, which possesses its own degree of difference. Unlike benign head formations, if craniosynostosis is not treated, it will only become worse and pose a threat to the sufferer.

What are the signs of craniosynostosis?

According to the Mayo Clinic Staff, the marked features of craniosynostosis include:

1. Abnormal head shape—the shape depending on the sutures that prematurely closed.
2. Unusual or absent "soft spot" on the baby's skull. This is also known as a fontanelle.
3. Although your baby is growing, the head is not. That, or the growth is slow and delayed.

4. Hard, raised ridges on your baby's skull. As the sutures continue to be affected by the locked skull, they change and spread in different directions.

5. Intracranial pressure is present.

Craniosynostosis is not immediately obvious, though it is congenital. The symptoms become more noticeable as the craniosynostosis progresses.

What are the main categories of craniosynostosis?

There are two: primary and secondary.

❏ *Primary* is when the cranial sutures become hard and immovable. This in turn blocks the brain from growing as it should, thus locking it in.

❏ *Secondary* is the opposite. In primary, the brain can't grow because of the fused sutures. But in this case, the sutures fuse as a result of the brain, which is not growing as it should, or the brain's growth halts altogether.

If craniosynostosis varies according to suture closures, what are some of the most common types?

According to the American Association of Neurological Surgeons craniosynostosis and craniofacial disorders page, there are five recognized types of craniosynostosis. They are:

❏ *Metopic synostosis*: closing of the metopic suture, which is from the top of the head down the middle of the forehead, towards the nose. Trigonocephaly ensues, causing a triangle-shaped skull that points at the top and causes the eyes to bunch too closely together.

❧

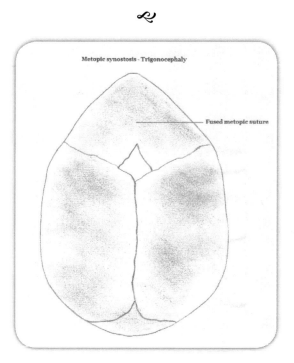

❧

❏ *Sagittal synostosis*: This causes scaphocephaly. As with Patrick, the head grew longer instead of growing in all directions. The forehead elongates, and the skull cannot grow in the left or right directions. This is common in males, and is the most common form of craniosynostosis.

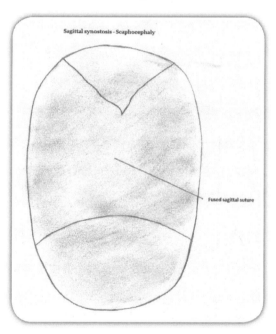

❑ *Lambdoidal synostosis*: premature closure of the lambdoidal suture, between the occipital and parietal bones. This is the rarest type, and it is marked by a raising of the ear, flattening in the closed suture's area, and the skull sloping sideways.

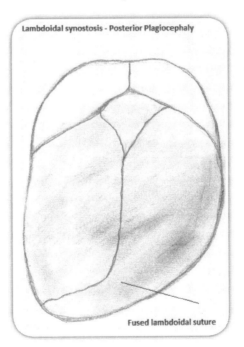

Lambdoidal synostosis - Posterior Plagiocephaly

Fused lambdoidal suture

- ❑ *Coronal synostosis*: by the ear and sagittal suture, which goes from the soft spot to the end of the head. The coronal suture, which extends from ear to ear over the top of the head on either the right or left side, closes. This closing causes anterior plagiocephaly—or a flattening on one side of the head (as can happen with sleeping on one side of the bed). This can raise the eye socket, deform the nose, and cause vision problems as a result.

- ❑ *Bicoronal synostosis*: the coronal sutures on both sides of the head are involved (coronal suture being the suture that separates the parietal bones from the frontal bones). When the coronal sutures close early, this leads to a condition called brachycephaly. The appearance of brachycephaly gives the child a flat, elevated forehead and brow.

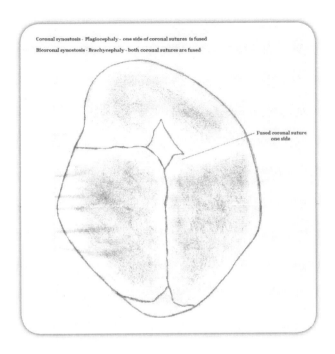

Coronal synostosis - Plagiocephaly - one side of coronal sutures is fused

Bicoronal synostosis - Brachycephaly - both coronal sutures are fused

Fused coronal suture one side

In general, craniosynostosis is more common in males and occur in at least one of every 1,000 live births.

Beyond the five types listed above, the type of craniosynostosis is further broken down into these two types: nonsyndromic and syndromic.

❑ *Nonsyndromic Synostosis*—includes a single suture or multiple sutures with no other syndromic features.

❑ *Syndromic synostosis*—usually several sutures are closed, and other syndromes are present. The most common syndromes are Crouzon, Apert and Pfeiffer syndrome.

What are these "syndromic features" that can accompany craniosynostosis? Crouzon, Apert, and Pfeiffer syndromes are examples. They are the other types of cranial syndromes that are important to distinguish from the aforementioned craniosynostosis types. Information provided by the American Association of Neurological Surgeons Craniosynostosis and Craniofacial Disorders page.

❑ *Apert Syndrome*: Apert is characterized by skull deformation. This means the skull can be unusually long, wide, or raised in a certain areas. The nose may shift, the eyes may bulge, and it's not unusually to have sunken areas in the face. Additionally, this affects the lower area of the face: "The upper jaw often has a narrow arch with an open bite and dental crowding. Other possible clinical problems include hydrocephalus, moderate hearing loss, speech impairment, and acne" (2005). This syndrome is very rare, affecting one infant in every 100,000 to 150,000 births. One of the main features of Apert Syndrome is strangely the hand. The fingers' skin and tissue fuse together, on both hands as well as the feet. Even though the skull is affected, people with Apert Syndrome aren't stunted intellectually.

❏ *Crouzon Syndrome*: This syndrome, unlike Apert, is typically genetic (although not necessarily. Twenty-five percent of cases aren't due to family history). This is more common—one in 25,000 births. The occurrence of Crouzon syndrome is also more common in bicoronal synostosis. Those with Crouzon look similar to Apert's patients. In both situations, it is preferable to operate within the first few months of age and before one year old. According to AANS, "Aside from facial deformities, other possible clinical problems include hearing loss, dental crowding, nasal airway obstruction, a v-shaped palate, and a condition of the cornea called keratitis" (2005).

❏ *Pfeiffer Syndrome*: As with the aforementioned syndromes, Pfeiffer Syndrome is caused by premature fusion of skull bones, creating a misshapen head. Additional symptoms include: "abnormal growth of these bones which leads to bulging and wide-set eyes, a high forehead, an underdeveloped upper jaw, and a beaked nose." It's not unusual for children to have dental and hearing problems as a result. Shortened fingers (brachydactyly), fingers that bend away from each other, and webbed phalanges (syndactyly) are other giveaway characteristics of Pfeiffer Syndrome. Like Apert, this is a rare syndrome that occurs about once in every 100,000 babies and is caused by gene mutations.

Pfeiffer Syndrome is broken down into three further types: Type one fits the above description and doesn't hinder the lives of those who have it. Their intelligence is normal. Type two is extreme, along with type three, but what distinguishes type two is that there are more fusions in the head, creating a marked cloverleaf-like shape. The latter two types pose more dangers to the brain, causing developmental problems, and are distinct from type one in that the nervous system is more heavily affected.

What causes craniosynostosis in the first place?

Usually, the cause is unknown as it is very difficult to pinpoint the answer to this question. However, in hereditary cases such as Patrick's, the cause is an abnormal chromosome or gene. The FGFR-2 protein (FGFR stands for fibroblast growth factor receptor) tells immature cells when to become bone cells and when to stop changing these cells. The protein producer cannot do its job correctly in craniosynostosis, being unable to send a signal to stop bone production. Thus the bones fuse prematurely, causing later bone growth abnormalities.

What are the typical complications of craniosynostosis?

The major complication of craniosynostosis, and the one that poses the most danger, is intracranial pressure. This prevents the brain from growing as it needs to because it's trapped under the prematurely closed skull. The Mayo Clinic staff outlines the complications of intracranial pressure as follows:

- ❏ Blindness
- ❏ Seizures
- ❏ Brain Damage
- ❏ Death (rarely)

Another possibility is facial deformity. This also presents a list of complications including:

- ❏ Upper airway obstructions, compromising your baby's ability to breathe
- ❏ Lasting head deformity
- ❏ Speech and language development issues

And, as one could imagine from a deformity, a low self-esteem results. These are complications no mother wishes to hear. They are dangerous and frightening. That's why it's essential to catch the problems earlier on and become aware of craniosynostosis to begin with.

What are the tests used to diagnose craniosynostosis?

Because the signs of craniosynostosis are visible to the doctors' eyes—elongated skull, raised bumps, points, etc.—they can decipher that way, along with feeling for bumps and ridges along the sutures of the skull. Besides that, radiological devices narrow down what type of craniosynostosis is as work, which sutures closed up, and how (and to what degree) the brain is affected. X-rays, CT scans, and MRIs show the details, which also determine which type of treatment is necessary, whether surgical or not.

How do you treat craniosynostosis?

Depending on the severity, the sutures involved, and presence of a syndrome, craniosynostosis can be treated in a variety of ways, but universally it is treated with surgery. If it's just a mild case, the child may require no treatment. Or, the doctor may prescribe a medical helmet. Most children require a surgery to better ensure a normal appearance and to relieve intracranial pressure.

Chapter 3
Deformational Plagiocephaly

"**M**ommy, I wanna hold my new baby brother!" An older sister might say. If the mother acquiesces, she will take great care in making sure the sibling supports the head and is very gentle with it. "Don't press on his head," the mother may say. This is because a baby's head is very malleable. This means the baby's skull is very soft and flexible and tends to deform very easily in the back and front, and also easily widens on the sides.

Many cultures, as far back as centuries, molded babies' heads in different shapes for vanity purposes. The Aztecs were well known for changing their head shape so it pointed in the back. We can still find many groups that still practice head molding (wrapping bands around babies' heads or placing babies on flat headboards) to recognize members of their own tribe or to identify status within the group.

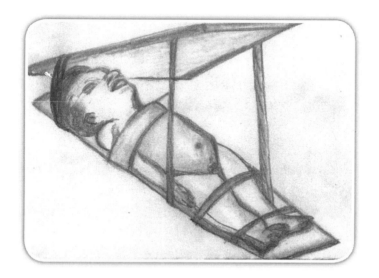

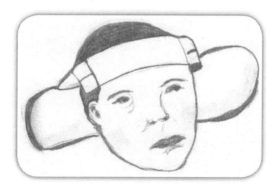

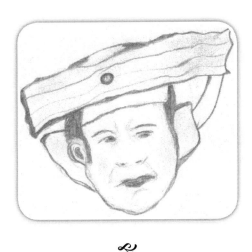

From different works of art, we can assume that cases of premature cranial sutures were present as early as centuries B.C., in ancient times. Head shaping was a prerogative of the upper class in Egypt, and it created an ideal of beauty and a mark of social status that was imitated for thousands of years (Favazza, M.D. 1996). This is because of the famous example of the Egyptian king Akhenaten, who was born with a very distinctive, elongated head shape. In ancient Egypt there was no knowledge of craniosynostosis, and so Egyptians tried to shape their infants' heads using bandages to produce a similar shape to that of the king. Nowadays we assume that King Akhenaten was born with craniosynostosis.

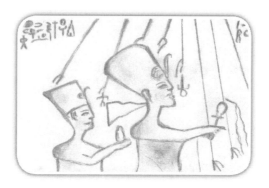

King Akhenaten

Because the baby's skull is so soft, many parents use this to their advantage by taking an active role in their babies' head growth. They are able to do this by laying the baby in different positions in the crib. The left and right side of the head should be symmetrical. Rather than laying the baby in the same position, such as on their left side every night, the parents may switch their positions so the head isn't molded to be too flat on one side. They are also careful about laying the baby on its back every night. However, the American Academy of Pediatrics recommends that babies sleep on their backs to prevent SIDS—sudden infant death syndrome. This is because if babies sleep on their stomachs or sides, they cannot get as much oxygen than if they laid on their back. This leads to otherwise healthy babies dying suddenly in their sleep. This warning is truthful and important, but at the same time it contributes to a rise in the flattening of babies' heads in the back known as *Deformational Plagiocephaly*, or "Flat Head Syndrome." This isn't craniosynostosis, but it is similar and can be a contributing factor to its onset.

Again, it is hard to describe exactly what a normal baby's shape should look like (and normalcy is defined by culture, as stated above), but generally the right and left sides should appear to be nearly identical. If pressure is applied to the same spots of the soft baby's skull, the head shape becomes misshapen. The different types of head shapes that result from this pressure are shown below.

❑ *Deformational Plagiocephaly* occurs when the back of the head on either side becomes flat.

⍋

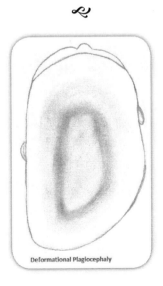

Deformational Plagiocephaly

❑ *Deformational Brachycephaly* occurs when both sides of the back of the head become flattened.

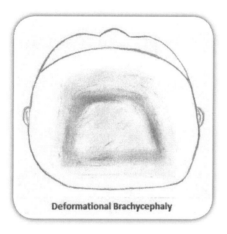

Deformational Brachycephaly

❑ *Deformational Scaphocephaly* involves a head that has a long appearance with flattening on both sides.

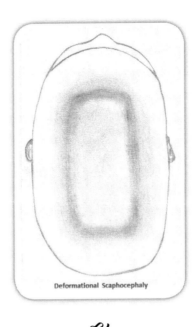

Deformational Scaphocephaly

What are the potential causes?

1. Among premature babies, the cause is often spending an extended period of time in the Neonatal Intensive Care Unit positioned in the side.

2. Torticollis, or the tightening of one or both of the neck muscles, is a culprit, and causes the baby to turn the head in one position, which then causes flattening of the same side of the head.

3. Multiple-birth pregnancies, such as twins or triplets, causes crowding, which affects head shape.

4. Intrauterine pressure, caused by unusual positioning in the uterus or the large size of the baby.

5. Sleeping position—too much time on just the left side, right side, or back.

6. Overuse of swings, car seats—as much as we all love them, including myself, these are a no-no for usage over long periods of time. A baby needs space for natural movement, and being kept in a swing or car seat does not allow them this freedom.

How to Prevent Deformational Plagiocephaly:

Deformational Plagiocephaly can be corrected almost always without surgery, but it's preferable to prevent it in the first place. In order to do this, try these tips:

1. Place babies on their back while they sleep to prevent SIDS, but alternate the head position from right to left and vice versa.

2. Give them frequent and supervised "tummy time."

3. Use swings and car seats less.

4. Rotating the position of the baby crib or the baby in the crib.

Different treatments for Deformational Plagiocephaly:

There is no evidence that DP causes brain damage. The sutures of the head are not fused as with Craniosynostosis, so the developing brain can grow without restrictions. Even if DP doesn't affect mental development, social development can suffer. A kid with a different head shape is subject to taunting—we know how mean kids can be to each other. That is why many parents seek treatment.

Treatment Options

1. Prevention: in cases where only the back of the head is flattened and the face looks symmetrical, carefully rotating and positioning the head away from the affected side will help. Once the babies start sitting on their own, the flattening may resolve itself spontaneously.

2. Molding helmet: if the front of the baby's head looks asymmetrical, simple positioning will not help. Usually babies under one year of age can be successfully treated with a custom-fitted molding helmet, which is worn twenty-three hours a day.

3. Surgery—In severe cases and older kids, the surgery might be the only treatment option.

The Importance of Tummy Time

Tummy time is a great preventative measure to avoid plagiocephaly. But what exactly does "tummy time" entail? According to the "Tummy Time Tools" article provided by Orthomerica Products, tummy time is:

❑ Any activity that keeps your baby from lying flat in one position against a hard, supporting surface

❑ Anytime you carry, position or play with your baby while he is on his belly (Coulter-O'Berry et al. 2006).

It's also fun and suitable for babies of all ages to prevent stiffening of neck muscles, promote development and strength of these muscles, and place equal pressure on the ever-changing, malleable infant skull.

There are plenty of ways to incorporate tummy time at home. Each everyday activity, such as diaper changing and playtime, can and should involve the tummy. Here's a list of ideas:

❑ When changing your baby's diaper, change the baby's position, rolling him or her from side to side. It also helps to talk to the baby from different sides as you do this.

❑ Place your baby on his or her stomach, facing its toys. This will help develop muscles for crawling and will further encourage the baby to look up and around at its surroundings.

- ❑ Lay down on your back with your baby resting on your stomach and facing you. This makes for good snuggle time.
- ❑ Carry your baby facing away from you, alternating the hip your baby rests on.
- ❑ Towel dry your baby on its tummy after a bath.
- ❑ Letting your baby rest on your lap on his or her stomach. You can burp them this way too, or burp them by standing them up, leaning their stomach on your knees.

When babies aren't on their tummies, there are other methods for avoiding deformational plagiocephaly. When a baby must be on its back, make sure the baby's head is turned toward each side, alternating when possible. If you want to avoid Sudden Infant Death Syndrome (SIDS) and lay the baby on its back, you should move the baby's head toward the left side one night, then on the right the next night. While a baby is against a hard surface—for example, a car seat—then it is recommended that the parents roll a towel to wrap around the baby's shoulders and head. This will keep the head from falling to one side.

Even if a parent follows all these suggested guidelines for tummy time and balancing head pressure, plagiocephaly can still strike—it's quite common. Under these circumstances, you would ask your doctor about the possibility of helmet treatment.

Helmet Treatment for Deformational Plagiocephaly

The STAR Cranial Center of Excellence staff works to mold the head to its ideal condition. With 1 in 5 children suffering head malformations, STAR Cranial Center of Excellence staff uses cranial remolding orthosis and is "the most widely prescribed cranial remolding orthosis in the world, treating more than 50,000 babies since 2001." They utilize a laser to make the most precise measurements for helmet production, which is what they used in Patrick's experience. On top of that, they provide precautionary materials in hopes of eliminating the problem of head malformations entirely—those that can be prevented. Guides, such as pamphlets and videos, are provided to raise awareness of aforementioned "supervised tummy time," and this company works with hospitals to ensure they are available.

If this is the route taken to fix your child's skull, the STAR Cranial Center of Excellence web page provides the timeline of treatment as follows:

1. Pending the scanning of your child's head at the pediatrician's office, your child should be fit for a helmet two weeks after the visit.

2. Five days after ascertaining the perfect fit, the child will wear the helmet twenty-three hours per day.

3. The family and your baby should return one week later to make sure the fit is still snug and that there are no questions about that part of the process.

4. Depending on your baby's growth, you will return to the doctor every two or three weeks for resizing purposes. Due to different areas growing at different rates, specific, specialized adjustments to the helmet will occur.

5. If the baby is four to seven months of age, the treatment program will be anywhere from three to four months. If the baby is older, longer programs are usually needed. This can be done to a baby's skull up until eighteen months of age.

As can be seen, the process is not uniform for each baby. Depending on the nuances of the baby's skull, a helmet is tweaked to meet the specific needs of that particular child. Though it requires much precision and time and many visits, measurements, and observation, this treatment has been successful for 50,000 infants around the country. These centers boast locations from Texas to Florida to Maryland, and they use the most novel technology.

Diagnosis:

As with most imbalances, sicknesses, and issues, parents and relatives spot the abnormality first. If you spot anything that you suspect looks unusual, even if you're nervous that you're just imagining a problem or that the problem will fix itself, go to a pediatrician. From that point, the treatment is typically straightforward.

An experienced physician can usually diagnose deformational plagiocephaly through a physical examination; X-rays or CT scans aren't typically necessary, although they may be used (along with MRIs). Generally any malformations are typically noticeable to the doctor's eye.

Chapter 4
The Evolution of Surgery Procedures For Craniosynostosis Treatment

C raniosynostosis is universally treated with surgery. Premature closure of cranial sutures has been known to exist for many centuries, and as everything in the universe, the surgical treatment for Craniosynostosis underwent its own evolution too. Many babies died in past during the procedure due to complications arising from surgery or the anesthesia.

We all are very blessed to live during this modern time and benefit from the advancements in technology and research. All the doctors and surgeons of decades past built principles and a solid foundation for the work of today's surgeons. Dr. Jimenez took into consideration these important findings and results from the past, plus his own experiences, and introduced his less invasive Endoscopic Strip Craniectomy to treat Craniosynostosis in the world. This is the type of surgery that has been practiced for years now by many surgeons with excellent results.

As early as centuries B.C., *Hippocrates*, "The Father of Medicine," mentioned the importance of cranial sutures. In the sixteenth century, anatomy scholars identified what we now know as sutures, were aware of various suture patterns, and categorized the various deformities that ensued from premature suture fusion. In order, this era gained the "appreciation of suture pattern and premature suture fusion in a variety of configurations by *Hundt*, specific abnormal varieties of sagittal and coronal sutures by *Dryander*, and what would now be described as oxycephaly and brachycephaly by *della Croce* and Vesalius" (Mehta, B.S. et al. 2010). However, in the late 1790s *von Sommering* was the first to lay the foundation for our present understanding of Craniosynostosis and subsequent surgical and nonsurgical interventions. He knew the consequences of premature suture fusion and more clearly understood sutures' roles in skull growth.

Otto was the first to reason that premature suture fusion resulted from skull movement, more specifically expansion, after observing skulls in both human and animal life forms.

In 1851, German doctor and pathologist *Rudolph Carl Virchow* published a landmark paper in the history of this medical phenomenon that he termed "Virchow's Law." It stated that he observed deformities occurring as a result of "cessation of growth across prematurely fused sutures" with "compensatory growth" along non-fused sutures in a direction parallel to the affected suture, causing obstruction of normal brain growth (Mehta, B.S. et al. 2010). This was the first accurate and generalized principle applicable to all patterns of premature suture fusion. He was also the one who coined the term "craniosynostosis." Interestingly, he first wanted to call it "craniostenosis," or "narrowed or structured skull," but Sear encouraged him instead to call it "craniosynostosis," which "more accurately indicated suture involvement and encompassed all varieties of suture disease"(Mehta, B.S. et al. 2010).

In the early twentieth century, craniosynostosis finally became recognized as a syndromic deformity. *Apert* and *Crouzon* identified and grouped it along with almost a hundred other deformities of its time within the first twenty years of the century (such as their namesake syndromes mentioned earlier).

Moss was revolutionary in that he challenged the notion of sutures causing the deformity. He believed it was the skull plates. Supporting his theory were four points:

1. "Sutures were often patent at surgery, even when there was a high degree of preoperative suspicion of suture fusion;

2. There were characteristic abnormalities at the cranial base that occurred with certain suture fusion patterns;

3. Excision of the fused suture did not always improve the cranial shape; and

4. Embryologically, skull development occurred after cranial base development."

(Mehta B.S. et al. 2010)

Moss's theory was disproven later because surgeries that aimed at prematurely fused sutures solved the problem—not surgeries that abided by his theory. However, value is seen in his work because he showed that brain growth affected these sutures' abnormality.

Although understanding of craniosynostosis as it pertained to sutures and brain growth were increasing with time, surgeries were no simple matter. The risks were great, as such an invasive surgery potentially (and often) caused blindness, neurological and cognitive damages, and hydrocephalus, the phenomenon by which fluid fills up in the brain—primarily in infants, as would be the case in this situation—and causes irreparable brain damage.

The first reported surgical interventions for craniosynostosis were strip craniectomies. These were first performed in Paris in 1890 by French surgeon *Odilon Marc Lannelongue,* who performed bilateral strip craniectomies for sagittal synostosis (the most common physical manifestation of craniosynostosis). He also strongly advocated for release, not resection, of the fused sutures. A major concern for this era was that craniosynostosis was easily confused with microcephaly and would not require the same treatment. Another was that by the time a child was operated on, the complications arising from failing to treat the craniosynostosis in infancy took its toll on the brain. Neurological problems already plagued the patient.

In 1892, he was followed by *Lane* in San Francisco, who also performed strip craniectomy. The mother of a child reportedly approached Lane and pleaded to him, "Can you not unlock my poor child's brain and let it grow?" He decided to have the child undergo surgery. However, the kid died fourteen hours afterward due to complications from anesthesia.

Despite these isolated reports with limited data on the outcome, it appears that this technique was quickly adopted and used for treatment of craniosynostosis (Mehta, B.S. et al. 2010).

In the early twentieth century, many kids who have been operated for craniosynostosis were misdiagnosed. The studies stated that they more likely had microcephaly than craniosynostosis, and those with true craniosynostosis were treated too late after the disease developed. The surgery only served as a temporary fix because of fast reossification (re-forming of the bones).

In this time Abraham Jacobi, "The father of American pediatrics" reported high mortality (fifteen out of thirty-three children died) and publicly denounced the practice to the American Academy of Pediatrics, marking the end of the surgery for decades.

He famously said:

> The relative impunity of operative interference accomplished by modern asepsis and antisepsis has developed an undue tendency to, and

rashness in, handling the knife. The hands take too frequently the place of brains…Is it sufficient glory to don a white apron and swing a carbonized knife, and is therein a sufficient indication to let daylight into a deformed cranium and on top of the hopelessly defective brain, and to proclaim a success because the victim consented not to die of the assault? Such rash feats of indiscriminate surgery…are stains on your hands and sins on your soul. No ocean of soap and water will clean those hands, no power of corrosive sublimate will disinfect the souls.

(Mehta, B.S. et al. 2010)

Too often, the doctors rushed into the surgery and did not conduct the surgery with the deftness it required. The amount of death that occurred was astonishing, and according to Jacobi, this was the failed responsibility of the doctor.

After a lull in surgery performance, it appeared on the scene once more when Mehner removed an abnormal suture safetly and successfully. Quickly thereafter in the 1940s, strip craniectomies and suturactomies were once again widely accepted, thanks to *Faber and Towne*. They differentiated microcephaly from craniosynostosis and pioneered the concept of early intervention—before two months of age—leading to better functional and cosmetic outcomes. They had hoped that using new surgical techniques would guard against blindness and other complications that arise from craniosynostosis. During the next fourteen years, the death rate significantly decreased, provided that their advice of treating children as early as possible was followed. Since then, many types of procedures were developed and performed, most of a very invasive nature. Complications did ensue from the surgeries, despite the advances in medicine. Reossification of bones over time became a problem when artificial sutures were inserted in the skull, and this led to a need for cranial vault remodeling—another risky venture to be detailed later.

By the 1950s, medicine continued to improve, helping the procedures of blood transfusion, anaesthesia, and the other components present in craniosynostosis-related surgery. The death rate decreased; "Shillito and Matson reported only two deaths in 394 operations, a stark contrast to the results reviewed by Jacobi just decades prior" (Mehta, B.S. et al. 2010). By this point, Shillito and Matson urged for emphasis in other areas of treatment, such as paying attention to restructuring the facial deformities that arose from craniosynostosis complications. Paul Tessier was one of such people that they coaxed to focus on treatment of the ensuing facial abnormalities.

In the 1960s, Paul Tessier pioneered the latter procedures and is regarded as the Father of modern craniofacial surgery. He believed that, although this is a complicated procedure, it could be done with care and with the skill of a strong team. Lingering during this time was a need to assist older patients who were more advanced in the disease. Younger patients enjoyed safer surgery with more favorable results, but a need for treatment development in older cases arose (in order to avoid neurological damage, a large risk at that juncture).

Jane et al. recognized this and developed the idea that "the major cause of the global cranial deformity was compensatory overgrowth at adjacent sutures" (Mehta, B.S. et al. 2010). As a result, she and her team pioneered the pi procedure to treat the most common form of craniosynostosis, isolated sagittal synostosis. The sagittal, bilateral, coronal, and lambdoid structures are removed in this process, and the parietal bones are broken and moved to encourage sideways skull growth. The sagittal suture is used as a rod to hold open the parietal bones, and the frontal and occipital bones are attached to the parietal bones, reshaping the head overall.

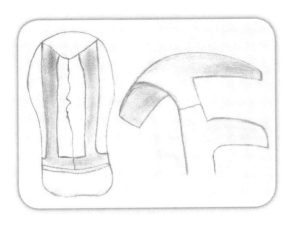

Illustrations of the pi procedure developed by Jane
and colleagues. Schematic of site and shape of
bone removed.

In the 1970s, the CT computed tomography was introduced,
which helped in better visualization of anatomical
deformities. This led to higher accuracy in diagnosis, which
was often a problem in the past, as mentioned.

The different types of craniosynostosis necessitated
different, specialized types of treatment. Let's home in on
these, as described by Dr. Jimenez:

1. Bilateral strip craniectomy: the resectioning of bone
    strips on either side of the midline from the coronal
    to the lambdoid sutures.

2. Wide strip craniectomy with bilateral wedge parietal craniectomies—or resectioning bone from parietal bones in inferolateral position to the squamosal sutures.

3. Sagittal craniectomy: removing sagittal sutures with piecemeal resection and replacement of parietal bones.

4. Subtotal calvarectomy and total vertex craniectomy: resection of calvaria top from coronal sutures to lambdoid sutures.

5. Midline craniectomy with occiput resection

6. Pi Procedure: the bones are resectioned to look like the Greek letter pi, transverse craniectomy at coronal sutures and bilateral paramedian strip craniectomies.

7. Total calvarial removal and reconstruction: resection of frontotemporal parietal and occipital skull. Then they are sectioned in many fragments and are replaced with plates and screwed in place.

One of the procedures chosen today in many craniofacial centers is Calvarial Vault Remodeling (CVR), known as *Traditional Surgery*. Dr. Jimenez has performed a large number of CVR procedures and has significant experience with this type of intervention. As he said, "Excellent results can indeed be achieved, but at significant cost to the patient," both financially and physically. A zigzag pattern is cut from ear to ear across the top of the baby's scalp, the skull is exposed, and the bones are removed, reconfigured, and reattached. Subsequent surgery is needed in most cases, and the skull may never look normal.

Other difficulties include the nature of the whole process. Surgical time is four to eight hours. Blood transfusions are universal. A long hospital stay, fevers, scalp and facial swelling, and pain are other hallmarks of the procedure. Other difficulties with Calvarian Vault Remodeling are improper skull reossification, palpable and visible "bumps and lumps," and accidental loosening of titanium screws, wires, and plates which have been found to migrate through the bone dura and into the brain, necessitating removal. Cyst formation was also reported near them. In recent years, these problems have been addressed by use of absorbable plates. No helmet therapy is needed after the surgery. The total cost is close to 60,000 dollars at this time.

New craniofacial surgical teams have popped up over time, and their preferred methods and techniques for surgery vary. The invasiveness and factors, such as blood loss, vary. They are sagittal strip craniectomies with circular occipital and parietal wedge osteotomies, keyhole craniectomies, bilateral parietal flap craniectomies, total vertex craniectomy, pi and reverse procedures, and other types of calvarial vault reconstructions. The smallest amount of blood loss is a few milliliters, and the largest goes up to a liter. Surgery time manages to stay eight hours or under for all procedures, and hospital time is at most one week.

In the early 90s, Dr. Jimenez and Dr. Barone have developed and successfully performed a less-invasive technique for the treatment of patients with craniosynostosis. They recognized the limitation of the approaches of the past century as: long operation time, the need for blood transfusion, and the need for repeated operations. They developed a procedure to decrease these problems called, "The Endoscopic Strip Craniectomy," which we will discuss in detail in the next chapter.

Chapter 5
The Endoscopic Strip Craniectomy: A minimally invasive technique to treat Craniosynostosis

With an endoscope in his left hand and surgical knife in his right, Jimenez watched on a monitor as he gently separated Bishop's scalp from the skull beneath.

Relaxed, his gloved hands quick and confident, Jimenez drilled two small holes into the scalp, then picked up his endoscope again and separated the skull bone from the dura, a protective layer of skin between the brain and the skull.

"How are we doing there?" he asked the anesthesia team. Above his mask, his eyes crinkled in a smile.

With the preliminary work done, Barone stepped in to open the fused suture on Bishop's head. She made a series of quick, crisp cuts with surgical scissors, first snipping a small wedge to enlarge the fontanel, then cutting a larger rectangle, about two-by-four inches, from the bony plate behind it. She finished with four narrow wedges that radiated off the newly opened suture, cuts that would help the head mold back into a proper shape.

The doctors finished their work by cauterizing the cut edges of bone tissue to stop them from bleeding.

Arranged on a cloth-draped tray next to the operating table, the skull fragments so resembled the shape of a turtle that the doctors and nurses paused to remark on it.

In fifty minutes, the entire procedure was over.

(Tumiel 2004)

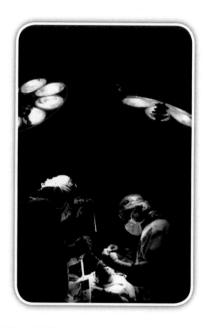

Dr. David F. Jimenez and Dr. Constance M. Barone performing Endoscopic Strip Craniectomy

As pioneers of this procedure to treat craniosynostosis, Dr. Jimenez and Dr. Barone believe that the high percentage of excellent results is due to a combination of *early* suture release—in patients younger than three months of age and helmet therapy. Nevertheless, very good results can be obtained, even with patients treated six or more months with appropriate postoperative helmet therapy.

Compare the characteristics of the Endoscopic Strip Craniectomy with Calvarial Vault Remodeling: It doesn't replace traditional cranial vault remodeling in older patients. By using endoscopes, instruments with cameras attached, two incisions are made in the scalp, depending on which sutures are involved. A strip of fused suture is removed. Surgical time is forty to fifty minutes. No or limited blood transfusions are needed. There are excellent results with extremely low morbidity and no mortalities. No swelling, no dural sinus tears, no infections, no cerebrospinal fluid leaks or neurosurgical injuries, the patient is discharged from hospital the next morning after surgery. The results are seen immediately.

A custom-made helmet is required for approximately one year following surgery. Postoperative helmet therapy can be divided into three phases: Phase I, Months one to two, when the first helmet is used to achieve a normal cephalic index; Phase II, Months three to six, when the second helmet is used to overcorrect cephalic index; and Phase III, months six to twelve, when the third helmet is used to maintain normocephaly and normal cephalic index. This technique decreases the overall cost. Cost is around 20,000 dollars at this time, plus each helmet costs approximately 2,000 dollars depending on insurance coverage.

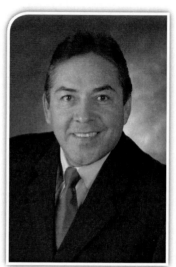
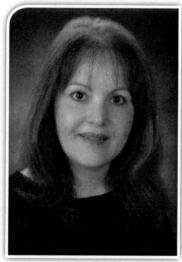

Dr. David F. Jimenez and Dr. Constance M. Barone's Autobiography

*"Anyone can make you smile or cry,
but it takes someone special to make you
smile when you already have tears in your eyes"*

Anonymous

Because most patients do require the surgical option for treatment, it's safe to assume parents wish for the least invasive, quickest, and most painless solution for their little patient. It's intimidating to think of your newborn going under the knife. That's why Dr. Jimenez's solution was preferable for me personally. To better know where Dr. Jimenez comes from and his credentials, read below (Material provided by UT Health Science Center Neurosurgery department page):

- ❏ According to UT Health Science Center's neurosurgery news page, he serves as the professor and chairman of the department of neurosurgery at UT Health Science Center at San Antonio and was recently elected President of Texas Association of Neurological Surgeons.

- ❏ He was previously President, Vice-President, and Secretary/Treasurer.

- ❏ He holds "twelve years of neurosurgery directorship and tenured positions as a professor in the University of Missouri-School of Medicine and University of Missouri Hospital and Clinics."

- ❏ Lecturing at over 250 meetings, he's a prestigious, traveling authority in the world of medicine.

- ❏ He has made special appearances on ABC's "Good Morning, America" and the Discovery Health Channel, a well-known doctor in the media.

❑ He serves as a member of the American Association of Neurological Surgeons, Congress of Neurological Surgeons, American College of Surgeons, and the American Clef Palate-Craniofacial Association.

❑ Philadelphia's Temple University, St. Christopher's Hospital for Children (Philadelphia), and the Albert Einstein College of Medicine's Montefiore Medical Center are his educational institutions that provided his training and studies.

❑ He and his wife, Dr. Barone, have traveled to the Philippines to treat children in unfavorable conditions who have craniosynostosis.

❑ His awards include: America's Top Doctors, Best Doctors in America, Top Doctors in San Antonio-Pediatric Neurosurgeon, the Continuing Education Award in Neurosurgery from the American Association of Neurological Surgeons and the Service Quality Award from University of Missouri Health Care.

His wife, Dr. Constance Barone, also boasts an impressive resume (information courtesy of the craniosynostosis physicians webpage):

❑ Professor of Neurosurgery at UT Health Science Center in San Antonio.

- ❏ "She received her B.A. from Smith College in Northampton and her M.D. from Mount Sinai School of Medicine in New York. She completed her general surgery residency at Temple University Hospital and her plastic surgery residency at New York University Medical Center" as well as training at the Albert Einstein School of Medicine.

- ❏ Diplomate at the American Boards of both Surgery and Plastic Surgery.

- ❏ Faculty member of the University of Missouri-Columbia School of Medicine from 1992 until 2004.

- ❏ Leader in plastic surgery and endoscopic procedures.

- ❏ Like Dr. Jimenez, she has a plethora of awards: Best Doctors in America awards and America's Top Surgeons in Plastic Surgery, plus she has been featured on Discovery Health, Good Morning America, Texas Monthly, San Antonio Magazine, SA Living, and Seventeen Magazine (2012).

- ❏ Along with Dr. Jimenez, she leads a team of experts who tackle craniofacial disorders, such as craniosynostosis.

Chapter 6
Post-Operative Helmet Therapy

B esides the surgical intervention chosen to combat craniosynostosis, the helmet therapy plays a huge role in the proper reshaping and healing of the skull. It's also the more long-term portion of the treatment—while the endoscopic strip craniectomy surgery tends to last around forty-five minutes, the helmet therapy is a months-long process and an equally integral treatment. Darren J. Poidevin, manager of the STAR Cranial Center of Excellence, offered information on his experience, as well as his more specific job descriptions, and the operations of STAR Cranial Center.

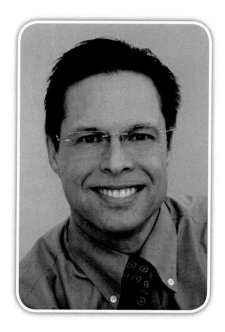

Darren J. Poidevin of Orthomerica

Darren J. Poidevin, CPO, LPO is a Licensed and American Board for Certification accredited Prosthetist and Orthotist. Darren is a graduate of Florida International University with a Bachelor of Science in Prosthetics and Orthotics and has 17 years of experience in patient management programs specializing in pediatrics, cranial remolding orthoses for plagiocephaly, and post-operative intervention for the treatment of craniosynostosis. While previously working with a National P&O provider as the

Practice Manager, Darren helped develop and implement the Cranial Program in San Antonio. Darren has trained and lectured across the nation as part of the National Orthotic team and Cranial Division. In addition, Darren has instructed on post-operative cranial remolding treatment for the Endoscopic Treatment of Craniosynostosis sponsored by the University of Texas Health Science Center at San Antonio, Division of Neurosurgery and the Plastic Surgery Department. Darren currently serves as the National Clinical Operations Manager for the STAR Cranial Center of Excellence located in San Antonio, working to ensure clinical excellence for multiple centers across the nation. Darren continues to treat patients and lecture nationally, with a specialization in cranial remolding orthoses for cranial abnormalities.

He wrote,

> The STAR Cranial Center Of Excellence (SCCE works closely with the area's leading pediatric neurosurgeons, craniofacial specialists, and pediatricians to treat patients with a variety of head shape anomalies including deformational plagiocephaly and craniosynostosis. SCCE is accredited by the ABC (American Board for Certification in Orthotics & Prosthetics). Our clinical staff consists of ABC accredited Orthotists and exclusively offers an unparalleled level of specialized expertise in treating infants with

plagiocephaly and craniosynostosis using the latest data acquisition technology, the STARscanner system. The STARscanner was the first scanning system approved by the FDA for the purpose of capturing 3D surface images of an infant's head shape. The STARscanner uses four Class I "eye-safe" lasers and eight cameras, which eliminates the need for plaster casting. The digital scanning process is the fastest, most accurate means of capturing the detailed information, taking less than two seconds to complete and accurate up to 0.5 mm. The STARscanner also provides a detailed comparison analysis report allowing referring physicians and families to visualize head shape changes before, during, and after treatment (See Item 1). The STARscanner's efficacy has been documented and published in the highly respected Journal of Craniofacial Surgery.

In San Antonio, Texas Doctors David Jimenez, Professor and Chairman of the Department of Neurosurgery in the School of Medicine at the UT Health Science Center at San Antonio, and Constance M. Barone, MD, FACS, a Plastic Surgeon and Clinical Professor in the Department of Neurosurgery in the School of Medicine at the UT Health Science Center, provide a minimally invasive endoscopic surgical treatment for the congenital abnormality craniosynostosis. I have had the honor and privilege working with Dr. Jimenez and Dr. Barone and hundreds of families from across the world. The STAR Cranial Center of Excellence has become an integral part of the multidisciplinary team and has helped develop the Post-Op Cranial Remolding Orthosis (CRO) protocols for patients being treated with the endoscopic approach for craniosynostosis.

At the SCCE in San Antonio, Texas I utilize the data acquisition of the STARscanner and use the detailed measurements report as a tool to assist in the thorough analysis an infant's head shape, as well as, to determine the appropriate modifications required in the Post-Operative CRO.

On Wednesdays, we participate in a craniosynostosis clinic, and offer a Pre-Operative evaluation, which includes collecting patient and family histories, a digital scan using the STARscanner, anthropometric measurements, and photographs. A copy of the scan is provided to the families, and then the Post-Operative CRO treatment goals and protocol are discussed with the families. The goal of the Post-Operative CRO, or any CRO, is to reshape the skull by using the infant's exponential brain growth. The CRO *does not* restrict brain growth, but with time, will redirect growth into void areas to achieve the desired head shape. A full report is given to Dr. Jimenez at the craniosynostosis clinic and the results and clinical findings are further discussed with the families. Surgeries are scheduled for

Thursdays, and patients are typically discharged from the hospital within one to two days. On Monday, the family and the patient visit our STAR Cranial Center of Excellence office for a follow up re-evaluation and scan. The scan is then emailed to Orthomerica, the manufacturer of the CRO, along with an order form detailing the patient's age, date of endoscopic surgery, involved synostotic suture, measurements and fabrication modifications for the Post-Operative CRO. The fitting of the Post-Operative CRO will be done within the next few days. The fitting of the Post-Operative CRO takes approximately one hour, which includes instruction on proper don and doffing, wearing schedules, and skin care and CRO maintenance. The family, patient, and I will again visit with Dr. Jimenez the following Wednesday at the craniosynostosis clinic to re-evaluate the patient and the fit of the Post-Operative CRO.

The patient will typically wear the Post-Operative CRO treatment for one year after surgery. Throughout the year, the patient will continue to check in with Dr. Jimenez and the STAR Cranial Center of Excellence, and depending on the patient's age and rate of growth, will require an average of three Post-Operative CROs.

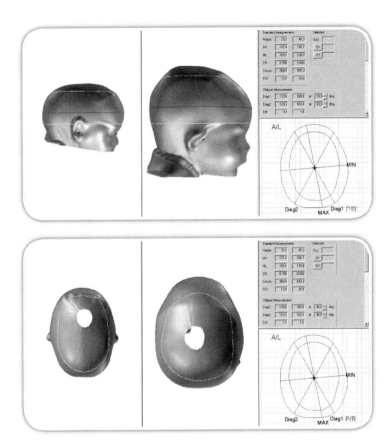

One cannot know about craniosynostosis and not admire the work that Dr. Jimenez and Dr. Barone contributed to the world of craniofacial surgery. He and his wife are both prestigious in their field and rightly so; the less invasive surgery technique is light years away from the dangers of craniosynostosis treatment in Jacobi's time. Thanks to him, my son's condition was dealt with swiftly and effectively. The unsettling concept of my son's brain being unable to grow is now just fantasy, a possibility of the past.

Part 2
Our Story

Chapter 1
The Blow

Anyone can hold the helm when the sea is calm.

Publilus Syrus

Patrick was two months old and a darling. I know all parents love to boast about their children and exclaim, "Our baby is the best baby ever!" All bias aside, Patrick truly was a dream baby. He was the happiest fella'—he never cried, he just sat and stared at us with curious cornflower-blue eyes. It took a lot to aggravate his calm demeanor. Our only complaint was that head of his.

During one of his regular wellness appointments, my husband and I decided to express our concerns about his head. "We noticed it's a little longer than usual," my husband, Casey, said about its alien shape. That was when it all started. The physician pursed her lips and said, "I'm going to go ahead and recommend a CT scan." My husband and I exchanged glances immediately.

"Is something terribly wrong?" I asked.

"Just to make sure everything is okay," she said.

I trusted it was just an added precaution. We set up an appointment and walked out of the clinic with Patrick in my arms. Without any suspicions or worry, I went home without knowing what God had in store for us.

My husband went back to work, Patrick and his two-year old brother, Charlie, were peacefully taking a nap, and I was lying on the couch trying to enjoy a few minutes of quiet. Two babies could really wear you out. I closed my eyes, soaking in the silence and the intermittent ticking of the clock.

Suddenly, the phone rang and interrupted me.

It must be my husband, I told myself. He always checks on us while he is at work. Lazily, I got up and found the phone.

"Hello?"

"Hey, mama," I heard my husband say. Ever since our kids were born, he has called me mama.

"Are you by the computer?" he asked. "I sent you an e-mail, go check it out."

"What is it? Can't it wait?"

"It's of huge importance to us. Just go look as soon as you can." His voice was stoic—I couldn't detect any lightheartedness. This all felt so very strange coming from my pleasant husband.

As much as I wanted to stay on the couch, I slowly walked to the computer and opened the e-mail. I clicked on the attached link and breezed through the Web site. Photos of babies scrolled down the page. Well, that's cute I guess, I thought. But I have my own cute baby. I wondered if he wanted another. But then I noticed their heads. At that moment, I didn't understand. Why was he e-mailing me all these photographs with little children who have some kind of head deformity? I shook my head confusedly.

I stretched and rose up to go to the couch and continue my rest during my sacred silence.

I didn't get too far. A realization materialized over my head like a threatening wall cloud, ready to strike me with lightening.

Bam! I bent over, feeling like I had been hit by a truck. My whole body started to shake, and I couldn't move another step.

Oh my God. Those three words circulated through my brain.

Oh my God. That was all I could think. Again and again. Am I dreaming, or do all of those kids in the pictures have the same head shape as our Patrick? Oh my God.

I felt a rock in my throat. I stumbled back to the computer and stared at the photographs; the tears warped the photos into what looked like warped watercolor paintings.

The message was received. Our little Patrick looked just like them.

When you come to the end of your rope,
tie a knot and hang on

Franklin D. Roosevelt

Chapter 2
The Search

Casey later gave me the verdict about his own realization. Stuck in post lunch hour traffic, my husband was driving back to work after Patrick's appointment. He tapped his fingers on the steering wheel to the radio beat and let his mind wander.

So curious, he thought about Patrick's head. I really hope everything is okay, as the physician said. Just double-checking, I'm sure.

Strangely, as a semi cut him off in traffic, the blaring truth slapped him across the face just as quickly as the blaring honk of the horn sounded.

Wait just a darn minute… His eyes widened and the hair on his arms stood on end.

As a concerned parent driving back to work, it clicked… he had a cousin who was born in the early 1980s with a condition that required surgery on his skull at around six months of age. My husband must have been around only six years old. So it made sense that he would have forgotten his cousin with the alien head, so remarkably similar to the one belonging to Patrick.

Thinking about it the whole way to the office, he rapidly whipped out his cell phone when he was finally in the building.

"Hello?"

"Hey Aunt Peggy, it's Casey," he said. His voice huffed and puffed as his legs pumped him to his office, where he could finally conduct much-needed research.

"Oh, hey there! Didn't expect a call from you today, how are you doing?" she asked.

"Well, the main reason I wanted to call was because of a question I had. I remember when we were little, our cousin had that head condition. I remember his head was longer and narrower. Can you tell me about that in more detail?"

"Well, let me see," she began, "it had to do with his head closin' early. Cr-something…cruh…long word, I'd have to look it up. Why do you ask? It's been ages since you've heard about this!"

"It has to do with Patrick." Casey rubbed his temples. "His head looks different from other kids', and it hit me that the last time I saw it was with Jessy. Patrick's head and Jessy's are identical."

"Oh, well then, let me look through some books and I'll get right back to you."

Each minute felt like an hour as he sat and twiddled his thumbs, waiting for his aunt to get back to him. Images of his cousin from back in the 80s floated in his mind. He remembered calling him a big head once, how his forehead was a lot longer than usual, and how bangs only accentuated that length. Definitely sounded a lot like Patrick. *Too* much like Patrick.

Brrrrrii—before the phone could ring all the way through one time, Casey grabbed it.

"Hello?"

"Hi there, Casey. Alright, I got it. Craniosynostosis. That's what Jessy had."

Cranio-hua!? Casey couldn't even wrap his head around the pronunciation, let alone the condition itself.

"Say that with me once. Cran—" he began.

"Craniosynostosis. The sagittal type."

"There's more than one type?"

"Search craniosynostosis online. I'll spell out each letter to you so researching isn't such a pain."

Before he knew it, Casey was desperately searching on the Internet for information on a previously unknown condition, a condition that certainly couldn't be affecting Patrick right now. Or so he hoped. The fact Jessy had it was all news to my husband, who thought he never heard that mouthful of a word in his life. He thanked my aunt, and quickly searched online for pictures, websites, and information. It was a surreal blur of information briefly passing over his eyes. Only one thing glued to his mind: the image of a baby's skull affected by craniosynostosis. Yes, it was Patrick alright. It was time to forward the information to me and shoot the email.

That was when I got it.

While looking at the pictures, it immediately became evident that our son was born with the same condition. Now we had to wait a few days for the CT scan to confirm it. I looked at Patrick cooing in the corner. He had a fine swathe of blonde hair that swooped to his five-head. Our minds were racing about the best options available to treat this otherwise healthy, handsome baby's deformed head.

"What happened to your cousin Jessy, Casey?" I asked.

"Nothing negative ever really 'became' of him," he replied. "He's just your everyday, normal guy, no problems."

"Well how did it affect his life? What's he like?" I had to know everything about the cousin who shared a fate with Patrick.

"It was so hard to remember he even had any problem at all because he's so normal. He plays a lot of basketball, football…he's got a good job, there's no issue. That should be a comfort to us, at least." We started thinking about Casey's cousin today who is a bright, athletic, successful person that never suffered any long-term issues from the condition. Our nerves were calmed, although we knew our son would have to have surgery. Our son going under the knife so early in life seemed unfair.

Everything that happened next happened very quietly without any unnecessary discussion.

For me, the hardest part at this point was how to share the news with my family. My husband took care of his side. They took the news solemnly, but lifted our spirits by offering their unwavering foundation throughout the process—both emotionally and financially. We truly couldn't have had a more solid support system. Now it was my turn; I had to call my parents, who lived overseas.

I picked up the phone and nervously rolled it in my hands. I didn't know what to say or how to say it. I still didn't know much about what was happening. Yes, we knew Patrick had craniosynostosis. Or did we? I still couldn't believe it was him. Surely our son is healthy—I glanced over at him again, sleeping on a fleece blanket. He had such a healthy rose glow in his chubby cheeks. He didn't seem to be in pain—he didn't fuss much. If anyone seemed to be in pain, it was myself. I was crying so hard all day I couldn't think clearly.

I had the worst scenarios in my mind.

What if this can't be fixed? That was not an option. And anyway, that's false. Jessy's condition turned out well; he was living life without hindrance.

What if this leaves him badly scarred? I imagined Patrick marching up to the front doors of his future kindergarten classroom, toting his lunchbox. Kids wouldn't even whisper as they would ask, "What's wrong wif your head?"

Patrick would be clueless. He would think this is just him, au naturale.

What if the surgery doesn't go well? What if there are complications? I needed to stop thinking this way. Tears already formed and were about to overflow onto my cheek.

What if…what if… These chaotic thoughts swirled in my mind. It was all completely maddening.

To tell the truth, I was scared to death for my little baby. Even if Casey's cousin turned out fine, what if Patrick was different? What if he had a more severe case? What if we didn't treat it in time? It was hard to even think about all that was happening. How could I dial the number and talk to my parents? To anybody! I had no idea. So, I just picked up the phone and dialed their number, still thinking about Patrick's little brain that needed to grow but had no room.

I was thinking about what could happen if we didn't help him as fast as fast as we could. Headaches, cognitive problems…unthinkable things. My fingers weighed five pounds each as I dialed each number.

As the other line was ringing, I felt the now-familiar big rock in my throat.

"Hello?" Mom asked a couple times. I tried to say something, but all I was able to get out was "Mom!" I yelped like a hurt puppy.

After that I just started crying; I couldn't say anything more.

It has been nearly four years since all this happened, and to this day, I can't think about it without getting tears in my eyes. It is so hard when your baby is hurt, you know it and feel helpless to do anything about it. Knowing its your responsibility to take away the hurt. It doesn't matter which illness it is, how minor or how major. Even a simple cold will turn your life around. You can't watch your baby suffering. There is no other pain like this.

After a minute, I took a deep breath and said, "Patrick will need head surgery," and started to cry again. I could feel my mom's tangible alarm on the other end of the line.

"What does he have?" she asked. I told her the name, and she, like me, had no idea what this long word was before the conversation.

"Shh, shh, it's alright," she murmured over and over. When I would stop to take a breath, my mother asked, "Could you let me know what this means, what is happening?" I took a shuddery breath and tried to put myself together. "Patrick has craniosynostosis. His skull closed early but his brain is still growing." This brought a fresh sting of tears. I know she must have felt hopeless being so far away and not able to be with us.

She assured me again and again that it would be all right, the way only a mother can do. Even though I didn't know what to expect yet, it felt good to know there was somebody I was able to talk to anytime, who was there for me, no matter what.

I took the opportunity to ask "why me?" to someone who would listen.

"Think about it, mom, I didn't drink or smoke. I did everything right," I said.

"Yes, yes. You've always been good. With Alexa and Charlie too. I wouldn't change a thing."

"And I even drank a ton of water this time around. I never do that!" As bad as it is, I prefer caffeinated or fruity, fun beverages. I asked her—and myself—over and over, "What did we do wrong? Whose fault was it?"

My mother didn't have the answers.

Later that day, I spotted Casey on the computer. I walked over and rested my chin on his shoulder. "Whatcha doing?" I mumbled.

"Taking care of it all," was all he said. As unlikely as that sounds, he was doing just that. I watched him as he Google searched the best craniosynostosis surgeons.

"Dr. Jimenez…look at these credentials." We took a closer look and saw that he consistently wins Doctor of the Year awards. I raised my eyebrows and nodded. Not a bad start. We explored craniosynostosis.net and were touched by the thank-you letters from patients. The testimonials mattered to us the most at that moment. The stunning part of the testimonials to us was that no one said a simple, "Thank you! Our son or daughter is doing great!" People expressed flowery speech from the bottoms of their hearts.

"This world is so blessed to have the two of you. You have touched our hearts and souls so deep—we are forever changed."

"You have truly blessed our lives and will forever be grateful. Thanks to you all for your love and compassion. You helped turn a tough circumstance into a wonderful experience."

"I couldn't believe how short the procedure and recovery time were—it was a miracle that I will forever be grateful for. I'm so glad I found his Web site—it changed my daughter & family's life."

Wow. These are no small compliments. The before and after photos were stellar as we saw tiny babies grow into smiling toddlers with no visible trauma. The last thank-you testimonial piqued our interest most though, the one about the procedure. That's what made my heart sink the most. Giving up my Patrick to sit on a cold operating table. I imagined myself waiting torturous hours for him. But the procedure was "short." Unbelievably so.

As we navigated the website, one claim in particular stood out to us: "A less invasive treatment," the site read. Not only that, but upon further research, we saw that Dr. Jimenez and his wife were the pioneers of such a treatment.

"If anybody knows how to do the treatment he helped start, it's gotta be him," Casey said. "Only the best for Patrick. Doesn't matter the cost."

The decision was easy as we read aloud his accomplishments: "Top Doctor in San Antonio... Best Doctors in America..." and then the philanthropy didn't hurt—he "treated disadvantaged children in the Philippines." The awards, the testimonials, and his appearance that just said he was a nice guy, all convinced us. Casey phoned Dr. Jimenez's assistant, Wai-Yee, that very same afternoon.

On the phone, Casey looked all business. His expression was statuesque and he nodded every few moments.

"Yes...photos? We can definitely do that. I will get that into you within the hour."

Pause, then, "CT Scan—yes, yes. On it."

He clicked the phone off and turned to me. "Where's the digital camera?" He asked.

"Should be in that drawer beside the computer," I said.

Patrick was snoozing lightly, lower lip parted and protruding a little past his upper lip, and he sure looked comfortable. However, Casey thrust open the drawer, whipped out the camera, and decided naptime was over. He gently rocked Patrick awake.

"Hey little man, time for a photo shoot." Patrick was still wide eyed and adjusting to daylight, so Casey gave him a few minutes before he had me position Patrick on my lap.

"Look, Patrick! A bird!" I pointed to the water fountain outside to try to glue Patrick's attention straight ahead. Casey got a few snapshots of Patrick's profile, then straight ahead. We didn't think we needed too many—it was evident Patrick's head was a perfect surgery candidate.

Right after that, Casey simultaneously uploaded the photos to email Wai-Yee and phoned the clinic for a CT scan as soon as possible. I was rather immobile with shock. Here I was, a crying wreck on the phone with my mother, unwilling to accept that our son has what he has, and that action needed to be taken. Then there's Casey, who deserves a bear hug for his "Let's get down to business" attitude. I truly am the luckiest woman alive—I mother three precious children and married an industrious husband who loves them just as much as I do.

Within the hour, Wai-Yee responded to our email.

Turner family—

Officially, according to Dr. Jimenez, Patrick is a surgery candidate. You were right when you noticed that the head is uncommon and matches with the craniosynostosis photos on our web site.

The next step in the process is getting the CT scan to us. Depending on when you schedule the scan, the surgery can fall on one of two days: this time next week, or this date one month from now. Dr. Jimenez runs on a tight schedule and this surgery only occurs once a month. Let me know of your plans.

—Wai-Yee, RN

Once a month…that's it? We could either haul our bums to Texas—where Dr. Jimenez worked—and get it done by next week, or wait thirty more days.

Wait thirty more days?

I could not do it; I was a wreck already. How could I sit and wait thirty days? It would kill me!

And what would it do to Patrick? I had a mental image of a cartoon-brain huffing and puffing and trying to lift the skull. The pressure of the skull on the brain gave the brain bruises and killed brain cells. Help! It shouted. I shooed the image out of my head at once.

"Luckily for us, the appointment I got for the CT scan is tomorrow," Casey announced, removing the pencil from behind his ear and writing a reminder on the calendar. As if we could forget.

"Oh thank God." I breathed. "We can just mail the CD of the CT scan overnight. Not a bad plan."

As a result of Casey's management skills, we got in for the September fourth surgery date. That meant we had a week to get the CT scan, take care of the hotel, plane tickets, rental car, find a Mary Poppins for Patrick's siblings, and get packed. We had such a lengthy to-do list for a while there. Ten days in Texas is a long time away if you're leaving two of your kids at home. But we did what we had to do.

"Why can't I go?" Charlie pouted as we started organizing our luggage, and he began circling my legs.

"Ah, Charlie, you wouldn't want to go. Hospitals are so boring!" I told him.

"Hopsittal?" Charlie repeated.

"It's where sick people go. It's where your toy doctor works every day."

Charlie tried to register this and shook his head. "I wanna be wif Patrick."

It broke my heart to leave my other baby at home, but Charlie would be an impatient wiggle worm the whole trip. I imagined him asking to leave during the many appointments we'd have, wanting to go to McDonalds, getting cranky and needing a nap, and all the typical twos' behavior. I would never put a two-year-old through that. I tried to lift his spirits (as well as my own because I didn't want to leave him).

"You get to play with Tricia, though! Auntie Tricia and you will have *so* much fun!"

At this, Alexa's ears perked up. She was thirteen years old and transitioning into a high schooler. As a result she always wanted to prove herself.

"I bet I could take care of Charlie, mom! I could do it."

"Alexa, it would be such a long time alone with Charlie. You have school."

"Yes, but…" Good point.

"And you don't want to have to cook every day, do you?"

"Ha, I can't cook." We laughed at this, remembering her last batch of chocolate chip cookies that more so resembled lumps of coal than dessert once they came out of the smoking oven.

The day before we left for Texas, I was more than a little frazzled. I dropped by the grocery store for some travel-sized shampoos and to buy the kids some snacks while we were gone. I probably shouldn't have driven. I don't know how I got to point B from point A. The details of the trip and the whirlwind of the week were quite dizzying.

Honnnnnnnk! A white truck zipped ahead before swerving in front of me.

"What the—" I furrowed my brow until I looked at the speedometer. Forty miles per hour down a fifty-five miles per hour road. Oops. I was thinking about Patrick and looking down at him in his baby seat. My mind gears turned in slow motion, and I suppose I subconsciously expected the whole world to slow down with me.

When I got home, I knew it was time to wake up. I asked Casey what needed to be done, but he, ever the manager, just presented me with a few slips of paper.

"What's this?" I asked. But the papers spoke for themselves. Confirmations of car rentals, hotel bookings, and all the details for our trip sat in front of me.

"Wow, Casey." I knew I had been distracted, but Casey was a speed-demon for just about anybody.

"Maybe I'm a little Type-A." He smiled. I then understood—Casey dove into the logistics of the trip because it helped him forget about the stress of our child's condition. That's not to say he wasn't already perfect in many ways in normal life. I never met someone so knowledgeable about vitamins and nutrition, nor so nurturing to his children.

I gave him a huge hug, feeling grateful for all he had done. If I had done it, it would have taken days longer— and we were running on a tight schedule.

The day of the trip, our real life Mary Poppins, Tricia, waltzed in the door early that morning with fifty pounds of luggage.

"Trissssshaaa!" Charlie bounded into her arms, and she dropped her body bags to the floor before planting a fat kiss on his cheek.

"Hey there kids! How are you doing?" She hugged Alexa next, but I just sat there cracking up. She looked like she was going on a trip to Hawaii, not staying with a couple of kids for ten days. Casey noted the same thing.

"I don't know that you brought enough stuff for your stay, Trish."

"Oh, come on now," she swooshed her hand in the air nonchalantly and gave her brother a hug. It felt so good to have family around us before we went on our important mission.

Patrick was relaxing in my arms, and Tricia walked over to give our trooper some love too.

"Patrick, you better be good for the doctor. No fussing," she said. She winked at me and I smiled. Obviously this wouldn't be a problem. He was so easygoing for his age.

"Call us if you need absolutely anything at all," I said as I showed her around the house, pointing to the kids' special treats and the vitamins. "It will be nice to hear from family."

"No, you call *me* if you need anything," said Tricia. "I'll just be entertaining two kids, so you keep us updated on Patrick. We all hope for the best." Patrick looked around the room, unaware that we were all gossiping about him. I was so relieved that he didn't and couldn't know what was going on.

After some logistics explanations, Casey looked at his watch and said we had better get ready; the taxi would be here soon. I hugged Alexa and Charlie about five seconds longer than usual. I would miss them, but I knew they would be okay and that we could leave them with Tricia without a worry.

"Have fun in Texas!" Alexa shouted as we walked down our house's pathway. As if there was much fun to be had in this situation, but I said thanks anyway.

As we drove off to the airport, the realization that this whole situation was actually happening crushed me like a too-heavy weight at the gym. We were going to Texas, and Patrick was having his procedure. I held Patrick progressively closer and closer to me the whole ride there. Hopefully he didn't feel suffocated. I didn't want to hurt him more than he already was.

To cheer myself up, I reminded myself that we received the best support we could wish for during this difficult time. The same minute my husband told his dad what was happening, my father-in-law offered us financial support, no questions asked. "Thanks for your generosity. We will do our very best to pay you back one day," said Casey.

"Of course," his father said. "This is our grandson. We will be there to support you guys with whatever you need. Take the money. It's yours."

This was a huge blessing. Because we went out of network and didn't wait for referrals or approval, our insurance didn't cover a cent. It makes me very sad because we later found out that patients from other states have had no problems with reimbursement, even though they went out of network. I know the insurance companies have rules to follow, and we didn't wait for approval, so the fault was fifty-fifty. But still, they should take time into consideration when making decisions about what to cover or not—for us, time played a huge role in the case. I don't understand all the stonewalling because the kind of surgery Dr. Jimenez performs costs far less than the traditional method. It was a cause of concern to me, so I decided to talk about it with Casey.

"What can we do, this is what Patrick needs, and we need to attend to his needs. For his benefit," said Casey.

Patrick was fast asleep on his first plane ride, thankfully. He was still in my arms, and I wasn't planning on releasing him.

"I know that. As if we didn't have enough stress, there's this money issue."

"Yes. But we can't wait for insurance, Mama. Dad is helping, and we got Patrick in very quickly. The sooner this procedure happens, the sooner he's well again."

Who could argue that?

Chapter 3
The Big Day

If you do not hope,
You will not find
What is beyond
Your hopes

St. Clement of Alexandria

As we soared to the ground, the city of San Antonio came into view through the puffs of cloud. We saw the winding river and lush vegetation. I should have felt relieved, but I clutched Patrick as usual, wanting to cry. I dreaded the moment I had to give Patrick to an impersonal doctor who viewed him as just another patient. Patrick's eyes would grow to magnifying-glass size as an unsmiling doctor snatches him from my unwilling arms.

The next twenty-four hours were filled with tears and studying. I told Casey we should familiarize ourselves more with the information before the procedure starts rolling. Back to the craniosynostosis websites we went.

We got ready for our first meeting with Dr. Jimenez two days before scheduled surgery. We came pretty prepared, knowing every detail about the procedures after studying

Dr. Jimenez's web site over and over. But we still had mixed feelings of course. Would this be a snooty doctor who spouted out facts like a dry textbook? Would he mind putting us at ease and answering all ten thousand of our questions?

We walked into the appointment wringing our hands and occupying our minds by playing with Patrick. We clapped his hands together and watched as his face lit up in a clumsy smile.

"Patrick! You're going to be so good for the doctor, aren't you? You're going to show him what a great, calm baby you are!" I said.

The same prayer raced across my mind: *Please God. Give this doctor wisdom. Take care of Patrick, and help this doctor know how to take care of Patrick as well.* We were entrusting this man with our most precious possession's life. Call it ambitious, but we hoped that this doctor shared the same immeasurable passion for our son's health as we did. Casey and I clasped hands and were mostly silent.

This abject fear and uneasiness dissipated the moment Dr. Jimenez entered the room.

"Tatiana, Casey. I'm Dr. Jimenez." He had a smile that went from ear to ear.

"Pleasure, sir," said Casey. Dr. Jimenez shook his hand heartily before moving on to Patrick and myself.

"Here's the little guy! Nice to meet you both." Dr. Jimenez swaddled my hand in his strong, leathery ones and squeezed. "Welcome to Texas, y'all."

He had a demeanor and a visible strength of character that helped my muscles relax for the first time in days. I think he could tell how taxing everything was for us.

"Let's get down to business and make sure we're on the same page," he began. He asked if he could see Patrick, and I hesitantly handed our son to him. As he explained the process of what's going on with Patrick's head, using Patrick as a visual, everything began clicking. He explained everything that I outlined in the "cranio-*what*?" chapter.

"Everything is making so much more sense," I said.

"Great! I know some of the words sound crazy, but it's easier to understand than people would think with a name like cranio-whoozit," he joked.

Patrick was still in his lap, but Dr. Jimenez held him close and comfortable. The way he took Patrick into his hands, holding him like his very own baby, I knew without a word we were at the right place with the right man. Not only because of the groundbreaking endoscopic technique that would be used to fix our son's closed suture on his head, but because of the man with the biggest heart I ever met.

Every minute more in to the talking with Dr. Jimenez I saw a warm, loving, and caring person with a passion for life and everything he does to make his little patients' lives happier. He's the type of man who you feel is a long, lost cousin: he is playful with Patrick as if he's a nephew, there are no inhibitions, and you feel there's a familial link because he's so genuinely interested in his patients.

"I'm confident this will be successful," he told us after our detailed discussion. "I was talking to my first patient the other day—he has gotten so tall. He's in high school now. He's playing soccer and sounds like a champ at it too. It's just always heartwarming to see how great their lives are going. All my kids, all the patients, are doing so well."

As we talked, we learned his own child inspired him.

"When Constance and I had our first, our whole perspective shifted. We now empathized with our patients' parents on a whole new level. These weren't just patients, they were *children*—it could have easily been ours, but we were immeasurably lucky that he was born as healthy as he was. We knew that the status quo of craniosynostosis surgical techniques had to move toward something less invasive, less stressful. Anything we could do to help the peace of mind of a parent, because we now knew just how valuable it is."

He talked with us like he knew us forever, like we were his best friends. He went through the whole procedure, explained every detail, talked about his first surgery experience, and the conversation flew so naturally that we ended up laughing and talking about California's weather.

"It's absolutely gorgeous there," I said. "We don't get cold winters. It's warm and breezy."

"This must have felt like a womb for you then," said Dr. Jimenez, and we laughed because it is so humid in San Antonio. "Probably extreme; like a jungle for you guys."

"No, actually, summers in Sacramento become deathly hot." I smiled.

"Either way, I'm jealous! It's time I tried surfing up there sometime."

"You'd want to go to San Diego then! That's where it's a good seventy-two degrees."

My heart was still heavy when I thought about surgery. But if anybody was going to secure a happy, healthy future for Patrick, I had no doubt it was Dr. Jimenez.

To see the rainbow, you have to face the rain first.

Unknown

On the dreaded day of the surgery, we got up pretty early—if we had slept at all, I would say. I sat at the edge of the bed, rubbing my eyes. The room wasn't completely dark—a faint hint of gray light crept in the room. Patrick put his hands on the sides of the baby bed and stared at me as if expecting something. He had slept all night, which I was thankful for, but Casey and I tossed and turned. Everything had to go smoothly. We hoped and prayed we'd have no surprises.

We were silent on the way there, still trying to muster energy from our sleepless night and find the strength to endure the day. The only sounds were our rental car's engine rumbling and Patrick's occasional ga-ga noises. My heart was already thumping like ominous footsteps of a doctor coming to cut Patrick's head.

By contrast, the pre-operation waiting room was packed with patients, old and young, waiting to be admitted for all kinds of surgeries.

"Maw maw, I want to go now!" cried what must have been a four-year-old. "I'm tired." His face was plum colored and streaked with frustrated tears. Two other siblings were pulling on a purple rabbit.

"Okay, okay yeah. Be sure to look on the patio. It could be there. I—be quiet, Josh. Hush. Oh, sorry—yeah, patio or upstairs in the attic…" rambled a nervous-looking woman on the phone.

Crunching on peanut butter crackers. Yapping business lady on a conference call. Snoring of a father. Other couples talking logistics and trying not to fall victims to suspense. The nurses on the phone and the shuffling of papers. The smell of disinfectant and antibacterial hand gel.

I heard the sounds but felt the stares as we walked in. Patrick was the youngest there and I noticed others looked at the car seat with Patrick in it as my husband was filing up and signing all the paperwork.

I must have looked pretty desperate and bad—once again right? My hair must have been matted in a dark mess and it looked like I received a bloody punch in the eyes. Sitting there so scared, I caught the attention of the whole room, I guess. I hunched my shoulders and wrapped my hands around my knees. "Think positive," I said to myself.

Suddenly a woman approached me and sat next to me.

"This room will drive ya crazy, I swear." She smiled at me. "I used to feel like it was my personal dungeon for the next few hours."

"You can say that again," I said.

"Is this the patient?" She said, looking at the curious Patrick.

"Yes. That's our little man." I swallowed a rough lump in my throat. "Patrick."

"He's so cute. How old?"

"Just about two months old," I said.

"Wow. I'm here with my husband, but I'm accustomed to young surgeries. Yeah, my two boys, Joe and Justin, had to have surgery at about age two. They underwent a couple surgeries they needed for quite a while. I was just relieved to get it done." Honestly I don't remember the all details of her story anymore, but now I know how nice she was as she tried to ease my pain I had written all over my face. You don't remember many details of life, but you never forget the assorted instances of kindness that you receive. Thanks, mystery woman.

After Casey filed and signed a pile of papers, we essentially twiddled our thumbs for some time. The suspense had an effect on me. I started deliriously saying my thoughts aloud.

"I feel like I'm walking on the moon."

"Now what does that even mean?" He gave a weak laugh. "I thought that was a good thing, an exhilarating feeling, to walk on the moon."

"There's a helmet on my head. That big bubble the astronaut wears. It's like my exhaustion, and everything that is outside of the bubble looks distorted and far away."

"That makes sense. I certainly feel the same way."

"It's like I'm wearing the heavy astronaut suit too. It's pulling me down because there's no gravity. It's dragging me down; my heart feels like it's dragging down. And even though we know every step of this procedure is proven to be safe, and we trust our navigator, Dr. Jimenez, anything can happen with the next step. Like walking on the moon." I feared we could metaphorically float into space, and before the next step I worried we wouldn't be able to land on the ground safely. The new terrain is different, and we were afraid. We wanted Patrick to land safely and continue on his "space adventure."

After awhile they called Patrick's name, and I was surprised to be relieved. It broke up my thoughts and the monotony of being trapped in my head and in the waiting room. We walked with him in to a pre-surgery room where they took his vital data.

Shortly two anesthesiologists walked in, and explained every detail of their part. I knew these were medical professionals—and there wasn't just one anesthesiologist, but two, so if they both agreed on the steps to take, they were undoubtedly the best measures for Patrick. A rock that had been lodged in my throat during this whole process sunk to the pit of my stomach when I thought about Patrick under anesthesia. It's dangerous enough as it is for anyone who isn't an infant.

The anesthesiologists left the room and were replaced by a plump blonde nurse. She had a kind face but was shrouded in a dark cloud as one of my new enemies.

When I found out a week ago back then that Patrick had Craniosynosiosis, I though this was the worst moment in my life.

I was so wrong.

I didn't know yet how painful it would be to put Patrick into a nurse's hands and let him go for the surgery.

I knew I had no choice.

I knew Patrick was leaving to get help.

I knew he was in the deftest hands in the whole world for the treatment of craniosynostosis.

I knew all of it; you could ask me why this was happening and if this was right for my son and family, and I'd respond with the proper logic. But at the moment when they took him, my heart swelled and caved into itself like a dead star.

Gosh, just breathe, I told myself. *He will be ok. You know it!* I was telling myself again and again, each time in greater hopes of its veracity.

Before surgery, we met Dr. Jimenez and his wife and work associate, Dr. Barone. She, like Dr. Jimenez, radiated with the warmth of a sympathetic smile.

"Hi, guys," she turned her licorice-colored head to us and walked over. "How are we doing?"

"Oh, you know, trucking through," said Casey. He managed a wan smile as Dr. Barone gave me a gentle pat on the back. Dr. Jimenez walked over with his hands in his pockets and looked at us.

"How about this," he said. "Don't wait in the waiting room. That's not a fun place to be. Doctor's orders: leave the hospital and get some coffee across the street. It's a good little local place."

"Coffee…" I murmured as if this were a long, lost drink from ages past. "Yeah, I think we could use some coffee today." Casey nodded and we thanked the doctors.

Funny how we listened to Dr. Jimenez without thinking about it. We just walked out of the hospital like two mummies and went to get a coffee.

I had just put my order in for an Americano when my cell phone buzzed. I patted my pockets for it and drew it out wildly fast.

"Hello?"

"Tatiana. This is just a quick update from the hospital to let you know the surgery has just begun. You will receive another call the minute it ends."

"Oh, okay. Thank you." I felt like a zombie but was glad for the continual updates.

Casey and I took a seat at a cushy red booth and looked around. Upbeat saxophone music emanated from the speakers; intermittent roars from the blender interrupted it. Local art covered the walls, and the disparate styles made the wall appear like a patchwork quilt that cozily enveloped our weary selves. The smell of coffee was cozy and familiar. It would be not only okay to sit here instead of the waiting room; it was, of course, preferable.

"Nice place," I said, making small talk. Casey nodded and sipped his black coffee. The bitterness of my Americano slapped me awake, but I also felt warm and alert.

We really didn't know what to talk about because one person—and one person alone—was on our mind, and that was Patrick. If anyone else entered our thoughts, it was Dr. Jimenez bent over Patrick in the operating room. After what seemed like a reflective stupor, I snapped out of it.

"Do you want to leave now?" I asked Casey.

He nodded. "Yeah, walking will feel good."

On the way back across the street, my phone started vibrating angrily in my pocket. *This is early. Has something happened?* I all but threw my coffee at Casey in the rush to pick up my phone.

"The surgery is all done! Come on up," said Wai-Yee.

Was this a joke? "Forty-four minutes! It must be Dr. Jimenez's record time!" She laughed and said, "Yeah, it's always quicker than everybody thinks it will be."

"What is it?" asked Casey worriedly.

"They're done!"

"Wait, what?" It didn't seem to register on his face for a moment, but he nevertheless also tossed his coffee in the trash and we raced up to the hospital.

Dr. Jimenez and Dr. Barone were already waiting for us with big smiles on their faces, looking like they just came back from a relaxing trip to the beach. I knew instantly that everything went smoothly and that Patrick was safe.

"Your son did great!" said Dr. Jimenez.

Since producing tears was on my agenda for a past few days, how could I break the pattern, right? So instead of saying something or asking something, here it was again, the ever-present, big rock in my throat and tears all over the room. Casey put his arm around my shoulder and we hugged.

"Oh, don't let me be rude. But let me introduce you to this random guy over here," said Dr. Jimenez. Thankfully my husband was there too so they actually had somebody to talk to. I just sat blubbering as always!

"This is a German neurosurgeon Dr. Hannes Haberl that traveled all the way over here to observe Patrick's endoscopic treatment. He was present during all of the surgery," Dr. Jimenez ushered to the towering man in the corner.

"Hallo," he said, vigorously shaking Casey's and my hand. I'm not going to lie…I kind of felt privileged that Patrick had two excellent neurosurgeons who watched over him during the surgery.

I shook the German doctor's hand and said nothing of course (you know my agenda right?) Gosh, I could have at least spat out *Danke Schon* or something, forgetting that I used to teach German language in high school before my boys were born. My tongue was tied, but hopefully he understood. Just in case, *Danke Schon,* Dr. Haberl, for being there for my son. My latest knowledge is that Dr. Haberl got home safely and is already practicing Endoscopic Strip Craniectomies in Charité-Hospital in Berlin.

Patrick spent a couple hours in the Intensive Care Unit, but later that evening they moved him to regular room because they needed room for new patients. It was a busy night for the Intensive Care Unit.

Seeing all the other patients covered in bruises, stitches, and swollen, I am telling you Patrick looked like he should not be there at all. No bandages, no bruises, no swellings, sleeping peacefully in the bed…only the cables and tubes all around him reminded us why we were there. You could hardly see the scar.

But exactly as we were told, after a couple hours—six or so, he woke up and acted like nothing happened. His blue eyes popped open and his face said, *Why am I here, Mom and Dad?* His cycle was predictable and alternated: Ate and slept, ate and slept.

There was always a nurse checking on Patrick. Not really necessary considering my eyes were glued to him from the second I saw him after surgery. My husband was relieved at the sight of him and instantly felt better.

"I think he's in good hands and he's doing really well," said Casey.

"We couldn't have asked for better doctors," I agreed.

"Well, I'm sure Patrick will be just as well in a few hours. What do you say you turn in for the night? I can wait here with him."

"Mmm…" I acted like I considered it for a moment, but my answer was clear. "No." Call it stubborn, but I call it being a mom. I wasn't about to let Patrick out of my sight. "I will be the one staying here."

For the night my husband went back to hotel room so he could get some sleep and pick us up the next morning. Of course I could not sleep—who would? But everything went smoothly; we got through the night and were discharged the very next morning. Sooner than I had anticipated.

Maybe you're thinking I am making it up, but if you see Patrick's picture the day after surgery, laying on the bed in the hotel room, you would not guess he just underwent such a serious surgery.

Dr. Jimenez worked magic. This seemed too easy for Patrick—he didn't cry once! Not one single time. Sure, he still must have been under the pain medicine from during the surgery, and we were giving him Tylenol and Ibuprofen rotating every three hours, but still, I could not believe how peacefully he rested next to me. After three days we skipped the Tylenol and kept giving him Ibuprofen, only lowering the dose every day.

Six days after the surgery, we went to an orthotics appointment for Patrick's first helmet. This appointment is scheduled for a couple days after the surgery to make sure all swellings, if there are any, have gone down. This way the orthotist can get the best measurements so the helmet will fit perfectly (you can read all the details about the helmet therapy in the next chapter).

In a day the helmet was ready and on the tenth day after the surgery we went for a check up. Dr. Jimenez checked on Patrick, took his pictures, made sure the helmet fit perfectly, and with that, we were good to go home with our brave "Little Helmet Man."

Going to the airport was like a game of dodge ball. I pushed Patrick so slowly that my hair must have grown two inches.

"This floor is rough, slow down," Casey reminded me.

"I thought I was going slow…but good plan."

Corners were particularly challenging.

"Let's just slow down…slow…slower…" Casey was directing me like a backseat driver, but I was eating it up and going even slower than he probably intended.

"Okay, Patrick, we're turning now. Hold your helmet on tight." I prepared him for each turn with a soothing voice—partially for my sake.

It was a brand new experience for us, carrying a baby with a helmet around the airport, all worrying not to hit any bump while moving Patrick around. Everything fared so fantastically thus far. Couldn't let it change now.

Once we travailed the airport and all its foes and all the obstacles, we were seated soundly in the plane. I was triumphant.

"We did it," I told Casey. "I felt crazy because I was such a nervous wreck, but we did it."

Casey smiled. "Yes we did. We can breathe easy," he said. "And hey, I might not have seemed like a nervous wreck, but I was."

"You? You kept so calm. Well, mostly."

"I did all my crying on the inside." We laughed now because seeing how Patrick had taken the surgery like such a trooper removed us from the pain of uncertainty before. As he slept on my lap, I noticed the sunlight falling on Patrick's head like a spotlight. Blessings, like the sunlight, fell on our son.

There are only two ways to live your life.
One is as though
nothing is miracle.
The other is as though
everything is a miracle.

Albert Einstein, German physicist

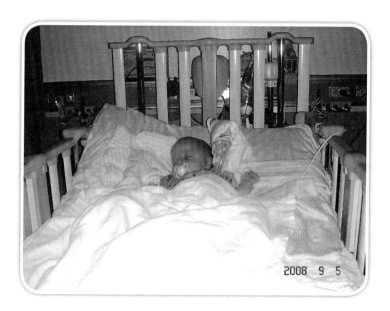

Right after surgery

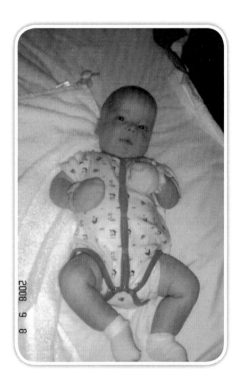

Four days after surgery

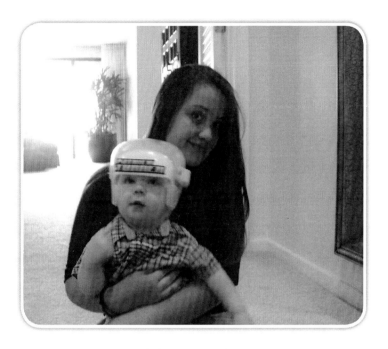

With my sister, Alexa

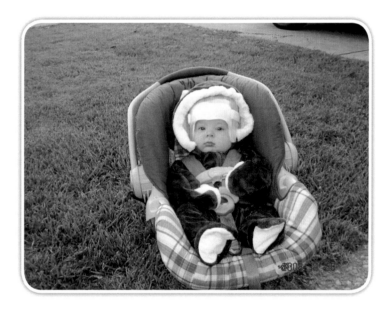

Going for a ride

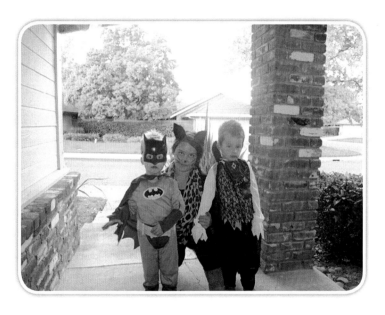

With Alexa and Charlie

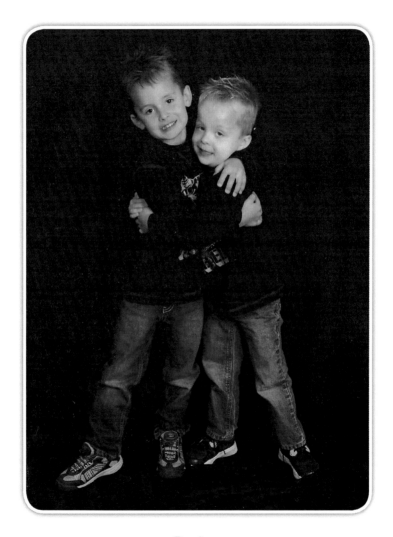

Brothers

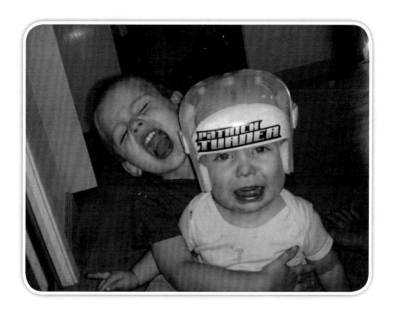

Brotherly love

Tatiana Turner

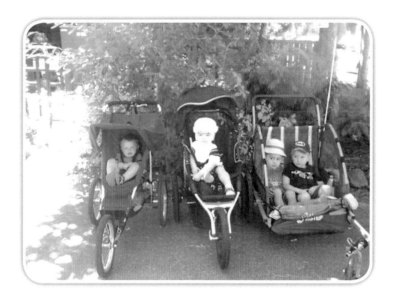

On vacation with my cousins

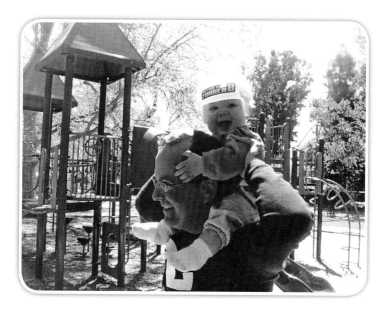

Me and my dad

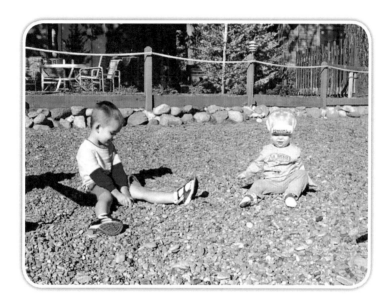

With my brother, Charlie, on the beach

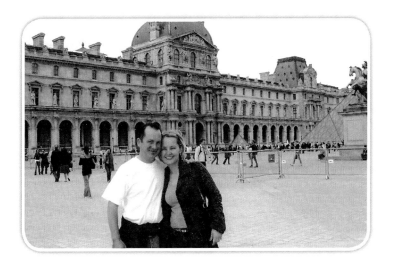

My mom and dad

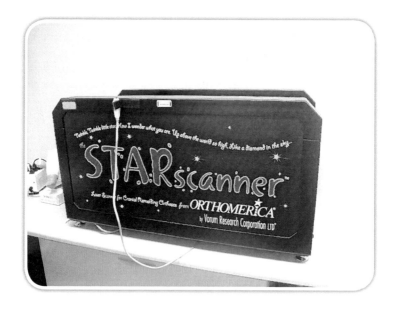

Starscanner from Orthomerica

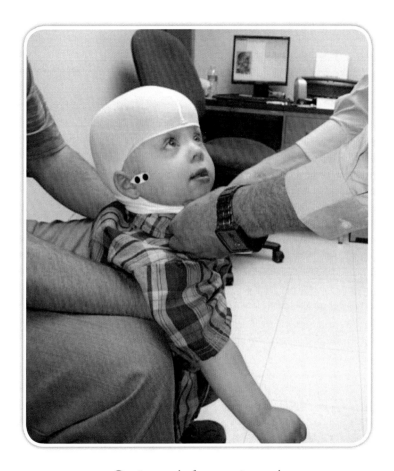

Getting ready for scanning and
measurements for a new helmet

Tatiana Turner

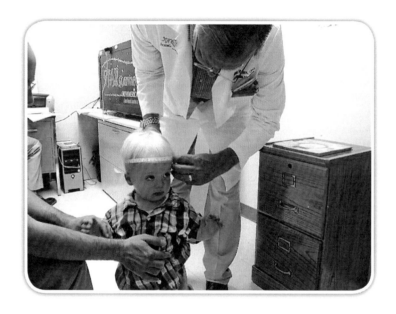

Taking measurements for a new helmet

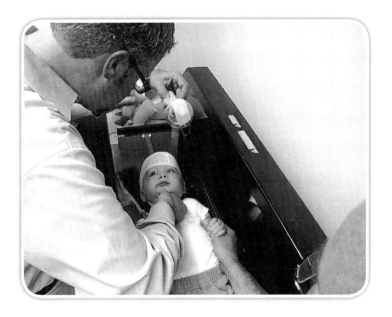

Patrick being scanned for a new helmet

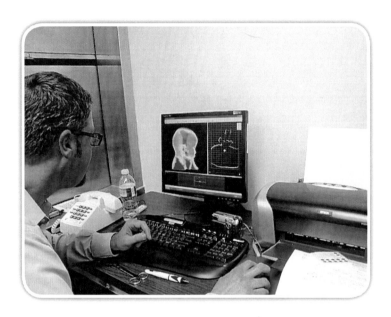

The scans are sent to the manufacturer right away
so the helmet can be shipped overnight to Texas

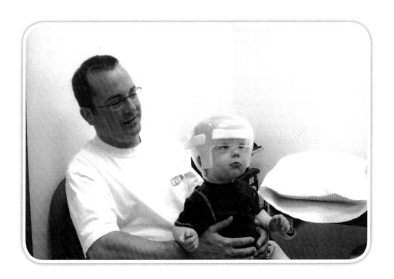

Patrick before his helmet was cut and fitted

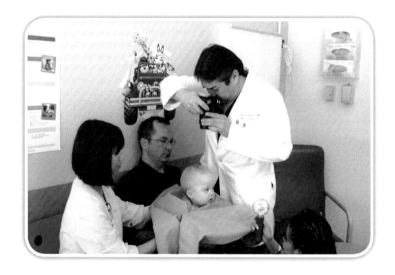

Dr. Jimenez and Wai-Yee taking head shots

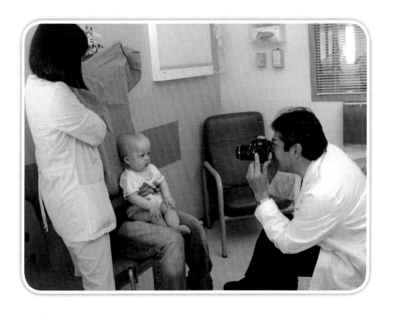

Dr. Jimenez takes photos of his patients' heads

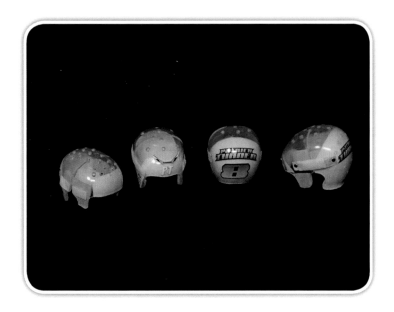

From the left: side, front, back, side

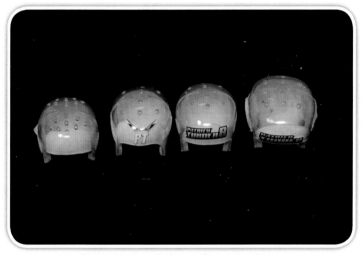

Patrick's four helmets from the front

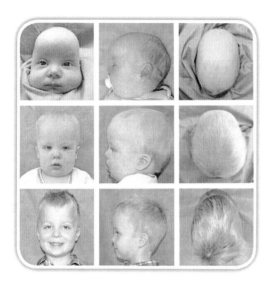

1st row - before surgery at the age of 2months
2nd row - at the age of 8months
3rd row - at the age of 3.5 years

Chapter 4
Post-Operative Helmet Therapy

Life may not be the party we hoped for, but while we are here we should dance.

Anonymous

As I mentioned before, helmet therapy is an important part of the whole treatment. The helmet not only protects your little one's head, but also helps achieve the best shape for the head by supporting the correct growth. The helmet is made according to the type of craniosynostosis that has been diagnosed. It is designed to apply pressure to areas of overgrowth and overcompensation while providing extra space for areas of restricted growth secondary to craniosynostosis.

In Patrick's case—sagittal suture synostosis—the helmet is padded in front and in back to slow the growth in those areas. Remember that he had a long "fivehead" and we needed his head to grow wider. The helmet succeeded. After its use, Patrick's head turned out to be a perfect shape. Doctors recommend that children wear the helmet until eighteen months of age for the very best outcome. Patrick was two months old when he underwent surgery, so we went through four helmets altogether.

Even though we were concerned at the beginning about how we would master all the manipulation with the helmet, it soon became a part of our daily routine with little or no problems. It took us a little while to figure out the best way to put the helmet on Patrick's head. He couldn't sit up on his own and couldn't lift his head yet. As every parent would be, we were worried to even touch his little head that just underwent such a serious surgery.

"Tatiana, hold Patrick," Casey told me. Bath time was a true test of teamwork, and thankfully for everyone, Casey had the most important role.

"Hey little helmet man, sit tight for me." Casey cautiously loosened the helmet and slid it off Patrick's head. Each day that we saw his head, we were more encouraged. He was slowly but surely looking normal.

"I'm so glad you're working the helmet. I'm always so worried Patrick's head is too delicate for my bull-in-a-china-shop touch," I said. For some reason I trusted him more than myself. I was still afraid to touch Patrick's little head. I just knew nobody could do it better than my husband.

"No problem, Mama."

"We appreciate it, Doc," I said. Casey, my husband, is our family "doctor." If anybody gets sick in our family, he will search and Google until he finds the best treatment for you—sound familiar? It is he who prescribes the medicine and takes care of the daily vitamins (if Casey says it's a good vitamin, you can bet it's the best kind on the market). Our kids assemble like soldiers every morning in the kitchen, and he can't leave for work until they ingest their daily dose of vitamins.

"Flintstones vitamins and omega-three gummy fish today, kids," he says while dispensing each one into the palm of their hand.

"Yummy, I want more," says Charlie almost every day. He thinks the gummy vitamins are candy like sour worms. That's how you know they're convincing.

"Are you sure you didn't miss your true calling?" I'll joke to Casey. "Health seems to be a priority right up next to cars."

"Nope, I work with, chat about, and manage the sales of cars all day long. That's perfect for me." He grew up in the dealership his grandfather built, so I think car-loving runs in his blood. But, still, he is the best caregiver one could wish to have at home. I can only thank his little obsession for health perfection this time that helped him find Dr. Jimenez.

After some time, we both became pretty good at manipulating the helmet. Patrick wore the helmet twenty-three hours a day. During bath time, one of us always washed the helmet with soapy water, especially during the hot California summer months when Patrick's head sweat so much!

"So much stink for such a small baby," said Casey. Believe me, I was wondering what stunk worse: the helmet, or his sister's sneakers.

Bath time was a feat of teamwork and finesse. Otherwise, we didn't have many problems with the helmet. There was one time when we got home from Texas and there was a little red mark on Patrick's head, which we thought would go away. Usually, in such a case, you are supposed to keep the helmet off for a day and the mark will go away. However, this didn't happen. I worried this was hurting Patrick's head, or that the wrong amount of pressure was affecting an area it shouldn't have. So, we mailed the helmet overnight to Florida, they fixed the helmet, and mailed it back overnight. We were lucky to receive such quick, excellent service.

I must admit that, as time went by, I started to like the multipurpose nature of the helmet. There were countless times that the helmet saved Patrick from bumps as he hit chairs or tables learning how to walk.

"I think the helmet giving Patrick a false sense of security," said Casey. Patrick had just smacked his head in the corner of the den coffee table, but he trucked onward on all fours. My husband still thinks this because Patrick bumped his head a lot after the helmet therapy.

However, he quickly figured out that without a helmet, bumps hurt!

Besides this, Patrick was a normal, growing boy. We could do normal activities as a family. Even going to the beach.

"Stay still, Charlie." I held him down so he would stop jumping up and down and from couch to couch. "You're going to need sunscreen."

"No," he whined. "It feels sticky."

"This kind won't be as sticky as it normally is." I shook the latest bottle I got, a new brand to soothe my children. Applying sunscreen on him was like bull riding—it was impossible to stay on. Charlie kept his eyes fixed on his bucket, shovel, and baggy of beach toys.

"Alexa, could you get Patrick, please?" Alexa just finished tying her hair in a messy bun so nodded agreeably. Patrick was spread eagle on all fours, making buzzing noises with his lips.

"Time for sunscreen for you too!" Alexa scooped Patrick in her arms, helmet and all. Unlike Charlie, Patrick didn't fuss a bit. If there was any discomfort, we were sure he could handle it.

All four of us piled in the minivan and drove to the beach, just a few minutes away. The sun and clouds looked idyllic; the clouds sat comfortably on either side of the sun like a pile of cotton balls in a preschooler's craft project.

Patrick peeked out the window every so often as if expected the sand and waves to appear any second.

We pulled up onto the gravel lot beside the wooden steps down to the beach. I lifted Patrick out of his seat, and Alexa and Charlie both bounced out excitedly.

"Don't run too far away from me, guys," I said, slinging the bag of beach toys over my arm. Patrick held out his dwarf-like hand and I took it, following behind the two oldest kids.

"Alright! I want to build sand castles," declared Charlie as we set down our towels.

"Make mommy a big one," I said, handing him his equipment. "Do you want to help too, Patrick?" Patrick looked like he belonged on the moon instead of a beach. His helmet was reminiscent of a space mission instead of a sand castle-building venture.

That helmet is going to stink so bad, I thought as I considered the ninety-degree weather. At least there was a sea breeze.

You wouldn't even know Patrick experienced a serious surgery. He and his siblings played together peacefully and without issue. One woman on the beach was looking at Patrick in curiosity though and walked over to me.

"Is he going to the moon or something?" She laughed facetiously.

"He has craniosynostosis." The woman's eyes shifted as if she were ashamed. I knew she had no idea what it was but supposed it must have been taboo. "Oh no…I'm sorry…" I now definitely had the feeling she had no idea what it was (why would she? I didn't know before either).

"Ha, no. It's perfectly fine. He's already had surgery to his head, and now he's wearing this helmet to make sure his skull is growing normally." I figured the hint would help her out.

"Well I'm really glad to hear it! He's such a brave baby for having already had a major surgery!"

"We know," I said. "We're proud of our Patrick."

Everywhere we went, people did a double take at Patrick and glanced at him longer than they would otherwise. But it was a good curiosity. I was always ready to raise awareness about craniosynostosis. Plus, they saw how mild-mannered our boy was, and how functional he was in every-day scenarios. He talked, walked, and developed normally in every other way. They learned about the condition but also learned it was treatable. And it awoke a desire within me to continue to acquaint people with this disease.

Chapter 5
Orthotics Appointments: What to expect

There will be bumps in the roads… but if you stay positive and believe that you can get through it, you will.

Savannah Rose Neveux

Mondays are many thing to many people, often simply the miserable commencement of a work week. For us, Monday was always the day when our check-ups in Texas began, starting first thing in the morning with an orthotics appointment.

As with any new doctor, the first trip was somewhat nerve racking. But as usual, the doctor—in this case, orthotist—put us at ease.

"It's nothing major. It's actually a pretty goofy process," he said. "It all starts with a sock." I looked at Casey funny.

This sock was specially-cut to fit Patrick's head(see photo), marked with little black stickers so the scanner could capture the best three-dimensional pictures needed for the helmet to be made. Then, the orthotist measured

Patrick's head manually and typed all the numbers in the computer.

"This way we will get Patrick's unique measurements to find the optimal helmet size and shape," he explained.

The scanners also vary. We went through two types of scanners during Patrick's helmet therapy. The one I liked better was a scanner that looked like a little gun, oddly enough (this type of scanner is discontinued in Dr. Jimenez's office). You would think that we would clench up at the idea of a gun pointing at our son's head, but it was neat and efficient. We held Patrick on our lap, and the orthotist scanned his head from every angle, effectively taking a three-dimensional digital image of Patrick's skull.

"The wonders of science and technology never cease to amaze me," I said to Casey when the image loaded on a computer screen.

The other scanner (the present choice in Dr. Jimenez's office) that our orthotist employed in our last two fittings is the Star Scanner (Orthomerica), which was a little trickier. This one is still used and yields great results.

The orthotist took us into a separate room, where we saw what looked like a giant microwave. "This seems like a giant MRI or CT Scan, and the process is very similar: Patrick will need to lay down on his back in the scanner and stay as still as possible, as still as a one-year-old can be at least."

"Good luck," Casey muttered.

"One way to make this easier is if one of you sits with him and tries to occupy him so he's still." Casey volunteered immediately, but I wanted to help too.

"We can use our typical teamwork," I said with a smile.

Casey held Patrick down and I tried to distract him with toys while the orthotist ran the scanner—again, teamwork. Most parents know the drill: you try to get the baby's attention or calm him down. You jump, sing, make faces, and do the craziest, most childish actions—yes, we did all of it.

"You parents are doing a great job, keep it up!...but Patrick still moved," said the orthotist after the first run.

"Darn it!"

"It's okay, hardly any of the kids have a great picture the first time. Maybe third or fifth time will be the charm," he said. Indeed, for us we never got a good picture the first time. Patrick was an otherwise agreeable patient though.

"I will say that he's one of the best little patients ever! He's very docile. I'm just glad there's no screaming or thrashing fit. That does happen quite often."

"So proud of you, Pato!" I said, holding his hand and waving it excitedly.

Once all the data were in the computer, the orthotist mailed the information to Florida, where the helmet manufacturer is located. They made the helmet that very same day and shipped it overnight back to Texas, just in time for our Tuesday orthotics appointment.

"No way," Casey said when the helmet sat before us, ready to go. "That's pretty spectacular! So fast."

"You have this down to a science," I agreed.

This appointment was a long one. Tuesday checkups usually took one to three hours. The helmet arrived in a condition that the orthotist needed to trim around the ear area and put in all the padding to make sure it fit perfectly. The process was very meticulous, but also very streamlined. Even with the precision involved to make sure everything was just right for Patrick, the organization and communications were impressive.

After an hour of putting the helmet on and off, hoping for a perfect fit, we were all pretty exhausted. I fed and changed Patrick in-between, walked around—it was just a long appointment for a little baby. It was long for all of us, really! The orthotist glanced up at us after fitting Patrick and said, "You do know this kid never cries, right? He's a rarity—it's amazing!"

"You're right. He never cried—not once. I think that's why everybody here likes him so much," I said.

"It does make the job go by a lot more smoothly. He's a good boy."

"Yep," added Casey. "We are very lucky parents."

We built a lasting friendship with Dave the orthotist. A big thanks to you, Dave, for all your patience. I must say that everybody from the hospital staff we met through our journey with Patrick was so nice and helpful that we almost forgot why we were there. We actually had a great time coming back for check ups and new helmets despite the entire situation. Genuinely good company makes a huge difference to ease the whole battle you are going through.

During this helmet phase of the process, some parents were very creative decorating the helmets, like our friend, Krista, from Oklahoma. We met her in the pre-operation room. Her son underwent the same type of surgery right after our Patrick, and since then we became friends because we were in the same shoes. Unfortunately for Krista, her youngest son—born two years later—was born with craniosynostosis as well. This is extremely rare and a terrible situation. On the bright side, she knew where to go, who to call, and that everything would be fine. She took the helmet to a body shop for a custom spray-painting job—so cool! I didn't realize how much fun decorating a helmet could be.

"Look at this photo," Casey said during one of our appointments. He pointed to photograph on the wall. It was taken during a birthday party for a little girl, wearing a helmet. What caught my attention was that every adult in the photo—probably twenty of them—were wearing the same helmet.

"Aww!" I smiled. "That's so precious. How sweet of them to do that for the little girl's sake."

"It's important to have fun with it. It's so much more fun for everyone to get creative: paint it, put stickers on it, have fun, enjoy."

And that's what gave us the idea to decorate the way we did. We already had vague plans, but since we are not much in the way of artists, we just chose to put stickers on the helmet that we could change. Casey ordered a few with Patrick's name from a website that sold auto-racing accessories. No surprise, since racing is a big passion in this family. We slapped the sticker on Patrick's helmet, and the vibe of his helmet became a lot more "cool," we said.

"He's now an intense racecar driver," Casey said. Patrick's name was branded across the front of the helmet, looking smoky and sleek.

During our daily life, only a few people knew the real purpose of the helmet. Some would stare thinking who knows what, while others would stop and ask where to get one and what team it was for. This always made me laugh. On rare instances, someone came right out and asked, as I mentioned earlier. I used it as a time to educate the masses on the previously unknown condition.

On Wednesday, we met with Dr. Jimenez, who checked the fit of the helmet, examined Patrick's head, and took pictures and measurements.

"Gather around, parents. This is what a perfect fit looks like. The helmet is great, Patrick's head is moving toward normal shape, and everything in general is going smoothly. I can assure you that everything is perfect." And it always continued to be.

On our last appointment, when Patrick was about sixteen months old, Dr. Jimenez gave us good news. "The long-awaited day arrived," he said.

"We're done with the helmet?" I asked hopefully. We made the experience fun for him with the stickers, but now we were ready to move past it.

"Ha! Not entirely, but that's coming soon. Patrick only has to wear the helmet at night. During the day his head is free."

We looked down at Patrick, who probably only ever remembered life with the helmet. "You're going to feel so free," I told him.

I will be honest: once we took the helmet off during the day, it was impossible to make Patrick wear it at night. He now knew and embraced the freedom of sun and wind on his head. He felt the effect of the California heat combined with the stinky helmet, and it didn't feel as good as his liberation in the daytime.

"Please, Patrick." Casey and I tried to settle him down before bedtime and make him comply with the helmet. He shrieked and wiggled out of our arms.

"No!" As with a few other one-syllable words, Patrick knew how to wield this one. And his answer was resounding and firm. *No!*

"But Dr. Jimenez says you have to," I said, trying to reason with him as if he understood. Casey made pleading faces to Patrick to guilt him into it. But he was already too old and fought us every time we tried to put it on. Patrick's face crinkled up like a prune, and he resembled a tiny old grandpa.

"Let's just give up," said Casey. "We fight with him about an hour each night to get this on, and we're so close to finishing this treatment anyway."

"Are you sure?" I asked.

"We've been good before, anyway. I'm sure this one thing won't matter." Yes, this was the only recommendation we didn't follow, but I know (hope) Dr. Jimenez wouldn't mind if he read this.

Chapter 6
Life Impact

*We make living
by what we get, but we
make life by what we give*

*Winston Churchill,
former British Prime Minister*

Sitting in the airplane on the way back home from San Antonio after surgery, I was looking at Patrick, our little helmet man, peacefully sleeping in his car seat. I was feeling grateful, so grateful that no words could express the feeling.

So grateful for the couple that helped Patrick. Not just Patrick, but so many other babies on daily basis.

I knew they were aware of how thankful we the parents are, and how much we appreciate all their work to this day, but I couldn't stop thinking about how to let the whole world know about these exceptional doctors. Every time people asked about Patrick's helmet, I fluttered at the chance to raise awareness of craniosynostosis and the instrumental work of Dr. Jimenez and Dr. Barone. This loving husband

and wife deserved recognition for their teamwork on the miracle treatment they pioneered for craniosynostosis.

I knew that Dr. Jimenez and Dr. Barone received much acclaim since their first introduction of the less-invasive treatment for craniosynostosis in the early nineties. There have been many articles and interviews published, TV apprentices, and awards for "Best American Doctors," but the experience was so strong for me that I wanted to do my part too. Their smiling faces and invaluable assistance in my child's life stuck to me like glue.

I knew our adventure would not stop with Patrick's surgery, helmet therapy, or a thank you note—a thank-you note would never be sufficient to encapsulate their meaning in the life of my son and myself. Looking from the airplane window, passing cities and states from Texas to California, I wanted to knock on every house and tell people about the two special doctors I just met—their awesome team, the couple who dedicated their life to others in full. Not just their personality and compatibility with parents from all walks of life, but about their unbelievable treatment they pioneered and all about how the babies successfully thrive after surgery. My desire to rave about them and the whole experience circulated in my mind like a marquee over a theater. In spite of the terror of the situation, they converted it into something simple, manageable, and even interesting. I now fully understood why the testimonials on craniosynostosis.net were as zealous and heartfelt as they were.

Think about it like this. How many true geniuses are born in one century? I'm not just talking about someone who attains a 2400 on the SAT or passes every test with flying colors. I'm talking about analytical, dreaming pioneers. Not only does the person have the means and intellect to enact change, they know exactly how to do it and always think to the future. They have the ambition and work ethic that nestle nicely with their big dreams, prodigious skills, and genius. How many people impact the world immediately and perfectly? Right, not many. So what are your chances of meeting one? Not really big. No doubt Dr. Jimenez and Dr. Barone are two of the few in the twentieth century, the century I got the chance to live in! With their groundbreaking treatment of a condition, one that is a very distinct possibility in the life of an infant, and the revolutionary ease of treating it with as little complication as possible, they truly deserve the title of *genius*.

It is so important for every parent to be a good advocate for their baby while choosing the right treatment, and this little book should help them in early diagnosis that is so important so their babies can be treated same as our Patrick with less invasive surgery if, of course, circumstances allow. Babies in Slovakia, India, or Japan...all over the world. Dr. Jimenez has already treated patients from Brazil, Canada, Chile, El Salvador, Germany, Mexico, Saudi Arabia, Mongolia, Spain, and the United Kingdom. If this novel treatment spreads to every other corner of the globe,

I may not be here anymore, but I will surely do my part and put every effort in while I can to raise awareness of the condition and the treatment (and oh gosh, I have big plans). This little book is only the beginning.

An important concept to embrace is that you should always trust your instincts as a parent. Even with brilliant professionals around you, hold your ground as the main connection to your child. For instance, use parental instincts in circumstances such as ours—remember our insurance issue? We sought swift treatment instead of waiting around for insurance. The insurance will assist you and the doctor because he is close to you or in their network; in other words, they are minding their own interests, not seeking out the doctor who is the *best* fit for you. That is why it is so much of importance for every parent *to be the advocate for your kid* no matter what.

Trust your mother—parents' instincts are *real*. They are not just a word; you just feel it when something is not right with your child. It's a sixth sense, in essence. No pediatrician can feel for your baby what you as a parent can, even the best doctor in the world is not connected to the baby the way you are. There are phenomena in the world that cannot be explained, and this is one of them—magic maybe, but I believe it's a gift from God.

Searching online and educating myself while writing this book, I read many articles and parents' stories whose babies had to undergo traditional surgery to treat craniosynosostosis because they were diagnosed too late to benefit from less-invasive endoscopic surgery, or simply the country where they live doesn't practice this relatively new surgery yet. I chatted with some parents overseas, and they didn't have any idea about this new type of surgery. Nobody told them, and even if they would have, most of them would not have the ability to fly to the United States, mostly because of financial matters. I cried with them; I prayed with them, feeling their pain 100 percent. Seeing the picture of babies with heads cut ear to ear, with their swollen faces after they underwent the traditional surgery, pushes me every day to finish my project and be able to raise awareness about this condition. After all, I was a mother for the third time, living in the affluent United States, and reading every informational baby book to prepare myself for any possibilities during pregnancy and the newborn era. In spite of that, I didn't even know about craniosynostosis and sadly, nor do most people. If they did, and knew how to spot it early on, the emotional and physical pain of the diagnosis and following traditional surgery would diminish.

Let everybody know what to look for early, early enough so their babies don't have to go through such an intense surgery. Let everybody know that there is a better way to do it, a less invasive way. We did it and it worked! Since the early nineties, when Dr. Jimenez and Dr. Barone introduced this type of surgery, they treated hundreds of babies from all over the world, successfully treated them, with excellent outcomes. It's just necessary that the children get diagnosed *in time*.

Since early diagnosis is so crucial, I thought it was interesting to read about Dr. Braverman, who developed a course—now required at Yale and many other medical schools—to bring their observational skills to the highest level. They are required to go to an art museum. That initially sounds useless or unrelated, right? But in the art museum, they observe paintings for a fixed amount of time, and afterwards they describe what they have seen. A study concluded that the technique improves the students' power of observation.

I think this is an excellent training tool for all medical students to become doctors. So much of the craft involves analysis and examination, and we should want doctors who won't miss any sign of a patient's physical abnormalities, which can be unique to each person. They should be spotters with good observation skills.

Personal opinions aside, I believe everything happens for a reason, and everybody has a purpose in his or her life. I found my purpose thanks to the adventure I traveled with my son, an adventure with a happy end. That is what matters most.

A very happy end.

And I will do my very best, so every set of parents who will have to go through the same adventure as we did can write the same at the end of their own stories.

Time is changing very fast; we live in such a great time of speedy evolution. What wasn't possible yesterday is possible today or will be tomorrow. I believe from the depths of my heart that there will be more and more surgeons all over our planet year by year, day by day, who will believe in the success of this less-invasive surgery, put some effort into it, become trained, and will start to treat babies this way—a better way.

The Little Helmet Man—
Nonprofit Foundation

www.thelittlehelmetman.org

*We don't accomplish anything in this world alone…
and whatever happens is the result of the whole
tapestry of one's life and all the weaving of individual
treads from one to another that creates something.*

Sandra Day O'Connor

Since my journey with Patrick's craniosynostosis started, I've slowly but surely fed a fire within me to chase what I believe is my life's purpose. I'm working to start a nonprofit organization that would raise awareness about the little-known craniosynostosis and do our best to ensure parents know it exists, what signs to look for, and that their education occurs when their children are young enough to seek vital early treatment. The specific tenets of the organization are below.

Our Pledge:

❑ Raise awareness about Craniosynostosis. Medical professionals and especially parents need to be aware that Craniosynostosis exists, otherwise they will be oblivious to early signs of this condition.

❑ Sponsor workshops about Craniosynostosis for parents, medical students, and pediatricians.

❑ Explain every detail about the condition and the importance of an early diagnosis

❑ Develop and distribute informational pamphlets and brochures about craniosynostosis to pediatric offices, birth, and neonatal units in hospitals, parents' centers, and medical schools worldwide

❑ Provide financial support for families worldwide who decide to undergo an Endoscopic Strip Craniectomy.

❑ Cover the cost of surgery, travel expenses, and the helmet therapy.

❑ Sponsor Neurosurgeons from outside the United States to attend yearly international workshop about the Endoscopic Strip Craniectomy for the treatment of craniosynostosis, held in San Antonio, Texas, by Dr. Jimenez and Dr. Barone.

❑ Help neurosurgeons with any preliminary needs so they can start practicing the procedure in their countries.

❑ Publish articles in magazines about this condition and update information on a regular basis.

❑ Finance the translation of the book *The Little Helmet Man or Cranio-what?* in many world languages to better spread an awareness of craniosynostosis and the less invasive treatment for craniosynostosis to as many cultures as possible.

The world can and does change one person at a time. Each person I spread the word to is another victory. I hope that one day, no babies' heads will be cut open in the intimidating invasive surgery. More and more doctors will be trained in Dr. Jimenez's procedure, and hopefully children all over the world will have access to the simple solution that we were able to secure for our Patrick.

Be the change you wish to see in the world.

Mahatma Gandhi

Thank you

I really don't want to miss anybody, so here's a general "Thanks a lot!" to all of you, my family and friends, who helped us and kept their fingers crossed for Patrick throughout our journey.

To my father-in-law, Pat: We almost drained your account, but all that matters in the end is that Patrick is growing into a handsome, smart little man.

To Casey, my husband: Thank you for everything. The list would be too long if I detailed each one of your acts of service and love. Maybe I should just write a new book for you! You always say, "Not everybody has what we both have," and you once gave me a keychain that said, "Life is better lived together." Isn't that the truth! We made it through. Together. It was a piece of cake with you by my side, and I still carry the keychain with me.

To my parents and my sister: Without each of you, I wouldn't be who I am today. Thanks for inspiring me and supporting me throughout my every endeavor.

To my kids Alexa, Charlie, and Patrick, and nieces Marion and Emily: You make my days colorful and my hair grey, but that's fine by me because grey is a color too.

Wai-Yee, RN: You put us at ease with your remarkable ability to keep us calm and informed of how everything would go from the very first moment we talked to you.

It is difficult to express how thankful we are for your kindness, warmth, and ability to help facilitate all of the arrangements for our son's surgery. You were incredible throughout the entire process.

Darren: Thanks for your valuable contribution to the book. Helmet Therapy is such an important part in the whole process. Keep up the good job; our little friends need you.

To Ashley: Thank you for offering your input for this book and helping it all come together.

Special Thanks to Dr. Jimenez and Dr. Barone: To me, you two are the most significant, beautiful people to cross my path in the medical field; you made the whole ordeal as comfortable as possible for two concerned parents. Thank you for your hard work, love and dedication. In life, there are only few people who are irreplaceable for us, and you are two of them for each parent whose baby you save.

Thanks for being the caring, hardworking individuals you are. We will never forget your impact on our lives.

Endnotes

American Association of Neurological Surgeons, "Craniosynostosis and Craniofacial Disorders." Last modified September 2005. Accessed July 13, 2012. *http://www.aans.org/en/Patient Information/Conditions and Treatments/Craniosynostosis and Craniofacial Disorders.aspx.*

Coulter-O'Berry, P.T., M.S., P.C.S., Colleen, and Dulcey Lima, C.O., O.T.R./L. "Tummy Time Tools: Activities to Help You Position, Hold, Carry, and Play With Your Baby." *Orthomerica Products, Inc.* (2006): 1-6.

Craniosynostosis.net. University Health Systems for Bexar County and Beyond, "Our Physicians: Dr. Jimenez." Last modified 2012. Accessed July 12, 2012. http://www.craniosynostosis.net/craniosynostosis-physicians/.

David F. Jimenez, M.D., Constance M. Barone, M.D., Maria E. McGee, M.D., Cathy C. Cartwright, R.N., P.C.N.S., and C. Lynette Baker, R.N., "Endoscopy-Assisted Wide-Vertex Craniectomy, Barrel Stave Osteotomies, and Postoperative Helmet Molding Therapy in the Management of Sagittal Suture Craniosynostosis,"Journal of Neurosurgery: Pediatrics, 100, no. 5 (2004): 407-417, *http://thejns.org/doi/abs/10.3171/ped.2004.100.5.0407* (accessed June 12, 2012).

Favazza, M.D., Armando R. Bodies Under Siege: Self-Mutilation in Culture and Psychiatry. Baltimore: John Hopkins University Press, 1996. 62.

Genetics Home Reference, "Genetic Conditions: Pfeiffer Syndrome." Last modified July 9, 2012. Accessed July 17, 2012. http://ghr.nlm.nih.gov/condition/pfeiffer-syndrome.

International Craniofacial Institute, "Craniosynostosis." Last modified December 4, 2011. Accessed July 17, 2012. *http://www.craniofacial.net/conditions-craniosynostosis.*

Mayo Clinic Staff. Mayo Clinic, "Craniosynostosis: Complications." Last modified September 29, 2011a. Accessed July 17, 2012. http://www.mayo clinic.com/health/craniosynostosis/DS00959/DSECTION=complications.

Mayo Clinic Staff. Mayo Clinic, "Craniosynostosis: Symptoms." Last modified September 29, 2011b. Accessed July 13, 2012. *http://www.mayoclinic.com/health/craniosynostosis/DS00959/DSECTION=symptoms.*

STAR Cranial Center of Excellence, "STAR Cranial Center of Excellence." Last modified 2008. Accessed July 11, 2012. *http://www.starcranialcenter.com/v2/site.html.*

"Tummy Time: Fun activities that promote symmetrical head shape and help babies develop strong neck and trunk muscles." *Star Cranial Center of Excellence.* (2007): 1-2.

Tumiel, Cindy. "UNIQUE SURGERY GIVES LITTLE BOY NEW LEASE ON LIFE: Improving on nature when their son is diagnosed with craniosynostosis, S.A.parents must decide which type of treatment they should seek." San Antonio Express News, November 21, 2004.

The University of Texas Health Science Center—School of Medicine, "Department of Neurosurgery: David F. Jimenez, M.D., FACS." Last modified July 5, 2012. Accessed July 11, 2012. *http://neurosurgery.uthscsa.edu/display_faculty_staff.php?ps_id=12&pg=faculty_*and_staff.php.

Vivek A. Mehta, B.S., Chetan Bettegowda, M.D., Ph.D., George I. Jallo, M.D., and Edward S. Ahn, M.D., "The Evolution of Surgical Management for Craniosynostosis,"Neurosurgical Focus, 29, no. 6 (2010), *http://thejns.org/doi/full/10.3171/2010.9.FOCUS10204* (accessed June 12, 2012).